THE JOURNEY INTO NATURE'S WELLNESS:
Art of Living Healthy

THE JOURNEY INTO NATURE'S WELLNESS:
Art of Living Healthy

Olubunmi Ruth Akiboye

Contents

THE JOURNEY INTO NATURE'S WELLNESS

ART OF LIVING HEALTHY

DEDICATION

This book is dedicated to those who would like to consider nutrition as a path to improving their health. My testimonies will encourage others so much that no matter what situation they are in; they will be assured of the benefits of nutrition.

It is also dedicated to my wonderful family; especially my husband and two sons who have been of immense help to me.

I also include all friends and mentors who have worked with me to bring this book to success.

May God bless you all abundantly.

INTRODUCTION

There are two major reasons I am writing this true story of my life. Firstly, I wish to bring awareness to those who suffer from long term sickle cell anaemia. This condition is not the end of the world. Some people in life experience worse conditions than others however, I believe it is possible to still enjoy a fulfilled life. Secondly, this book will encourage sufferers to understand that you can improve personal well-being through living a stress-free life. More so, this book will restore confidence and assist others through their journey of recovery as I have experienced.

*The next paragraph discusses issues linked with sickle cell. *

Sickle cell anaemia is a blood disorder, characterised by red blood cells that assume an abnormal rigid sickle shape. According to **T.L.Savitt**, this abnormality in sickle cell was first recognised in 1910 by **James Herrick, at the Chicago college of Dental surgery**. Sickle cells decrease the cells flexibility and this results in their restricted movement through blood vessels, depriving downstream tissue of oxygen. The disease is chronic and is lifelong. Individuals are sometimes healthy but their lives are interrupted by periodic painful crises and a risk of various other complications, such as stroke, heart problems, ulcers, acute chest syndrome to mention a few. It affects nearly every organ in the body. In some cases, life expectancy is shortened both in male and female respectively.

The genetics of sickle cell may seem complex but in fact are simple. If two parents carry the sickle cell traits and have a baby, then that child will have 1 in 4 chance of having sickle cell disease. A recent statistical finding on 23rd October 2019 by the NHLBI (National Heart, Lung and Blood Institute) asserts that sickle cell disease affects about 100,000 Americans and more than million people worldwide. A new release reveals that NHLBI led Collaboratory research identified that bone marrow transplant can cure sickle cell disease, but are most effective in children, who have well matched donors. Experience shows people who have the trait of sickle cell display low level evidence of sickle cell disease.

In my case I was diagnosed with sickle cell from the age of three months. I had a full blown sickle cell (SS) and my parents did not have a clue of what was going on as I was always in and out of hospital. I was born in the United Kingdom in the 1950s. At the time, no one had a clue of what sickle cell really was or knew how to treat it. It is quite unfortunate that so many people with sickle cell died of the condition at the time before the medical world came to learn more about the disease. I went through life in pain, but today I thank God that I am still living, all to the glory of God. The medical doctors are doing a good job, but my Creator does better.

www.nhlbi.nih.gov/health-topics/sickle-cell-disease

I would love to share my experience with those who have sickle cell disease including people with long term diseases. It has been a long journey. So many people have lost hope in themselves. However, others have decided to carry on with life. Generally, I have discovered that we are a unique set of people, no one is the same, as we are all fearfully and wonderfully made by the Creator. In my opinion, everyone that has sickle cell has a personality of their own; we are therefore different from each other. God has a plan for everyone, if you draw closer to him.

According to **James 4:8:**

> *"Come close to God, and God will come close to you".*
> **NLT**

Before the conclusion of this book you would realise that we are all created for a purpose and we would all live to fulfil that purpose. Remember our bodies function in the perfection that God created it to function.

Testimony:

Only those that have been in the fight can tell about the victories. It is those that have been tried to the utmost that come out and tell you the story about their life. And it is these people that can tell how they rejoiced and what they can do to help others live a life of peace and success. No matter what, we would get to where we are going without looking back. There is a bright light at the end of the tunnel and I am heading for it. It is out of experience I write what is going on in my life, and how I got to a place where I could say I am living my life to the best by the grace of God.

Myth:

There is a misconception that those with sickle cell live only up to the age of 21 or 22. Then it raised to 44, but these are speculations because no one knows how long anyone would live except God who created us. My health was not stabilised until I got to a certain age. Initially, I did not have the correct treatment and the nutrition my body required. My other discovery was eating right and drinking a lot of water. There are little things in life which we do not take note of and these are the most important ones that build up our bodies. It took me half of my lifetime to understand that the food I did not like, were the ones that nourished my body, but I thank God that I realised in time and these foods changed my life completely.

Going through the journey of my life, I realised that sickle cell disease (SCD) had affected me both physically, emotionally and mentally.

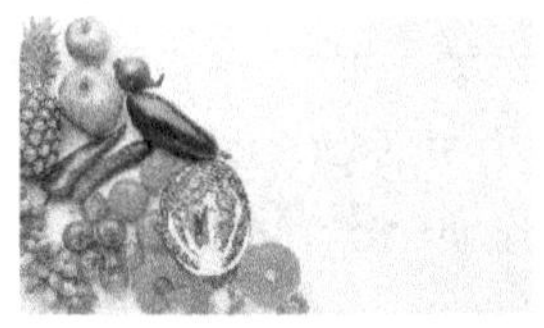

CHAPTER 1

The Beginning of My Journey

The whole problem started when I was born. As I was quite young, recalling everything is quite difficult. All I have are stories told to me by my mother and I was the child who never gave her any trouble at birth.

I was born with sickle cell anaemia, but then in the fifties no one really knew exactly what sickle cell was, till today there is no permanent cure. However, one could live a comfortable life by learning to manage various phases of crisis by doing the right thing. Everything was a guess, and there was no specific treatment for it. When I became six months old my parents kept on going back and forth to the hospitals in London where I was born. They did not have a clue of what was happening to me.

When I started nursery school, hospital visits were quite often and sometimes I was admitted. At the age of seven, the whole family went back to Nigeria. My health experience growing up in Nigeria was very rough. I was always in pain. It was dreadful. Once the pain started I rarely got any sleep for the next three days. I often cried myself to sleep. In those days there was nothing like morphine or oxynorm which numbs the pain, there was only paracetamol and codeine. Once the pain started Insomnia was the order of the day; crying myself to sleep. Most times I am given sleeping tablets that work for an hour and the pain starts all over again. Unfortunately, I suffered like this for a long time.

The pain was awfully consistent that I wished for a miracle to take away the pain immediately. Whenever I felt better, I'd have a feeling of resurrection. My mother would often appeal to me to lie down and get more rest whenever I joined my siblings to play. At the slightest opportunity,

I'd take a tour of the house inspecting to see if there was anything new I had missed.

My primary school years were not too bad, although when I started school it was a long way from home. We later moved nearer to my school. My siblings and I attended the same school initially but they were later moved to a private primary school which was further away from home. I felt a bit left out from the rest of my siblings, but the reason I was given was that close proximity would do me good during an emergency.

Furthermore, I remember faintly at times when my parents would want to take us out to funfairs or some interesting place. I would be so excited, only for my excitement to be shattered in disappointment as I may suffer a crisis a day before the outing thereby leaving me at the mercy of my grandmother. I was often teased by my siblings whenever they returned from an outing, although not in a bad way.

As a child, I often felt left out of so many things and that was because I could not participate in so many activities due to my sickness and I learned to appreciate each day and brace myself for any crisis. Playtime at school was always fun.

My mother was a designer of clothes who worked from home and this was because of my illness. I loved it whenever she was around. I always felt sad for reasons I can't explain whenever my mother went out. If I was ill she was always there beside me and That meant a lot to me and I cherished those moments. My grandmother always tried a lot of natural medicine like herbs that helped with pain and other symptoms. Some of them worked and some did not; they were bitter and I hated them. But some of these plants and herbs were particularly good. I was given a plant named **orin-ata** in Yoruba language (Zanthoxylum zanthoxyloides). The plant was a bit peppery and helped sometimes to keep the pain of the crisis away.

Towards the end of my primary school days, I developed eye problems, it got so bad that I could not see properly. I was referred to the University College Hospital in Ibadan. It was one of the good hospitals then, my late uncle worked there as a doctor. Once a month we would have to go to Ibadan for my eye check-ups. My parents and I had to stay overnight so I could be attended to at the hospital; I used to enjoy the journey and the hotels that we stayed in.

I ended up wearing glasses, with a double lens which was quite thick at the age of seven. At first, I had to wear them at night, (that was how bad my eyesight was) but later it was reduced to daytime only. This was another great mark in my life. I was wondering when this would stop, one minute it was my body, then it was my eyes, then my gall bladder and so on. But I continued with the journey, I never understood then what it was all about. I finally finished my primary school education, which on its own was a struggle but I managed to pull through. I remember that I used to pray a lot, I knew there was a God watching over me and that one day I will be free from all pain I experienced.

During the course of my sickness I fell for the myth which says that sickle cell patients do not live beyond 21 years. If one is not careful, one would live that trapped life and whenever I thought of the illness my heart sank.

Another hurdle came when I was to prepare for secondary school. I had mixed feelings. On one hand I was excited and looked forward to it, but on the other hand I was frightened of the future and how I will cope. Have you ever felt like that before in your life? That is the way I felt and was always looking for someone to encourage me, but there was hardly anyone around. In those days, there was not a lot of encouragement. It was just getting up and doing something. I had to face the common entrance examination before I could get into secondary school. My younger sister had hers done a year before and was admitted into one of the best secondary schools. Finally, I got a secondary school that admitted me, the journey of my life then continued.

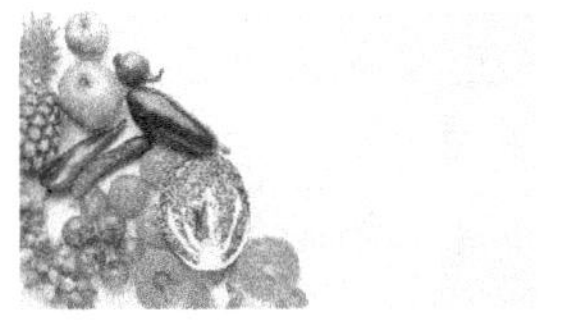

CHAPTER 2

Growing up with sickle cell anaemia

After the first stage of my common entrance examination I developed cold feet, asking myself if I will be able to succeed. There was no help, no advice, nothing hence I was left to think on my own. I was admitted into a secondary school I did not particularly like but I had no choice. Before I started my new school, my father passed a comment 'if you had done well you would have been admitted to a better college'. As a teenager, I was overly sensitive to words and that hurt me to the core. It made me feel incapable of doing things properly and not as good as others. But in my mind, 'I said that's fine'. I determined that whatever happens I will make the best of it.

The day I started secondary school, I was excited and was determined to try my best to move on in life. A few weeks later, I became ill and thought in my mind that I wish this crisis would go away. My grandmother and my mother tried their best with herbs but nothing worked. After a week I went back to college, I tried to catch up with my schoolwork, through the help of my classmates. I seemed to be the oldest in my class but that did not really bother me. I wanted to get my education over and done with, so I managed to finish that year with my classmates. As soon as I got to the middle of the third year, I began to get ill again and repeated classes. These were difficult times. It was so bad that I thought I would not be able to finish my education. I felt so weak that I wished for death. I summon up courage, that if I was alive now it means God has a purpose for me in life.

As I gradually finished my secondary school with great difficulty, I became more resilient. I hated exams as It was the greatest fight of my life, because without this I discovered I could not go forward in life. But after each exam; although I would feel a bit of relief there was always a nagging question of - if I would make it. My sister came out in flying colours in her exams and my father was so proud of her. My question now was what my own fate would be, at a stage I just switched off, I could not be bothered anymore as the stress was too much for me.

When my exam results came, I was devastated and wished the earth would open up and swallow me. I failed woefully, my mind began to race, my first thought was - What would I do? How can I face my family, especially my father? When I stopped thinking, the next idea that crossed my mind was to take my life! The thought was "no one would miss me anyway". As I settled for this wrong idea, I decided to take some pills and end my life. The stress was too much for me. I took the pills and laid down thinking I would go into the next world; wherever that was. I just wanted to be loved and encouraged, that there was more to life than this. No one understood me, I was full of self-pity and did not know what to do with myself.

God used my grandmother to save my life, she came in just in time to wake me up but it took her sometime. I could hear her voice in the distance but could not respond immediately. I gradually came out of the deep sleep but was so drowsy I could hardly stand. My grandmother was shocked! She kept on asking if I was okay in our native language, but I could not answer her. She knew there was something wrong, she could not figure out what it was.

However, I miraculously got over my suicidal attempt. As time went on, my father who was a legal practitioner and was quite busy, decided to get a teacher for me, to coach me so I could retake my exams. The teacher was so dedicated that it helped me to begin to improve in those subjects I was re-taking. He encouraged me a lot so that I began to understand those subjects I hated before. I found out later that he was a science teacher in one of the secondary schools. I took the exams and came out in flying colours especially in my science subjects, which I failed woefully initially. I was so ecstatic I began jumping for joy, as it was the first time in my life I had achieved something great.

After my joyous moments, it was time to choose my next journey. All my life I was interested in working in a hospital, taking care of people. So, I decided to go for a course either to be a dietician or physiotherapist. I knew it would be a great task health wise, but I was willing to do it anyway. After filling the form for admission, I needed someone to support my form and sign it. But when I went to those who could help me, like my family doctor and nurse, they told me they could not sign it because of my health. It was quite painful to give up my dream; I had no choice. As I was told to go for a course to be a grade 2 teacher, I thought not again; it was like changing the journey of my life to suit them.

The teaching journey of my life started as my parents wished as I began the course I had no clue about. It was a two-year course. Half way through the course I became ill again, I had another crisis. As usual three days went by before I could return to my education.

I was not a boarding student while I was in secondary school; I could not last long as a boarder, I think I lasted a year before my body began to complain. Funnily enough, I did enjoy the period I was in boarding school. I began another session of boarding at my Teacher Training College, this went on for another year. Later in the year, I fell ill again; this time the Matron of the college informed my parents to pick me up. The crisis started at night, I wished the pain would just go away but there was nothing anyone could do for me. I cried myself to sleep as the pain was so intense that it gave me a high fever. In the morning, a taxi was called and one of my classmates accompanied me home because I was too weak to travel back home alone as I could not walk. When I got home, I was surprised to see my father come out to the taxi. I thought the angels had visited him and that was the last time he did that.

Little did I know this illness called sickle cell could disrupt my life so much, in fact it got to a stage, I almost gave up. This was because nothing seemed to be working for me especially with my education as it took me ages to complete my basic education. I completed my education at the time and survived all turmoil by the grace of God. God loved me so much and he proved to me that I was fearfully and wonderfully made. God made all those with several illnesses beautiful and until we stop believing the lie of the devil we would not see ourselves as conquerors. I discovered that those with sickle cell are very intelligent, artistic and creative in all ways.

There has been so many lies going on around that those suffering with sickle cell cannot live past the age of 21 or 44. These are all lies of the devil. I am glad I have allowed God to defeat those lies in my life. The created cannot be greater than the Creator. If you listen to the deception of people for a long period, you would start to believe those lies. God in his infinite mercy has broken that chain. We are free to be the person God has created us to be. The blood of Jesus Christ has erased those lies from our lives.

Whilst in college, I was happy that I was coming towards the end of teacher training. I found the course interesting and enjoyed it up to a stage but it was not what I wanted for my chosen career. I was still bent on obtaining a career around health services, most especially Nutrition Science. I continued to search for jobs in a hospital like administrative work but found nothing. At the time, I required a reference or letter of recommendation but no one was willing to write one for me. So, I had to continue with the journey of teaching.

Eventually, I found a primary school near me and after all the formality of interview and filling of forms, I started work; teaching young children age range between 7 and 9 years old. It was not a bad job but it was not what I wanted. Not long after I started the job, I became ill again. This time, I nearly lost my life. The thought in my mind at the time was 'this is the end people were talking about'. I got well though.

We went for my great grandmother's funeral. I was between the ages of 20 and 21. Although I was fine and excited when we left for the village, on the day of the funeral, I suddenly became extremely ill. It started with an extremely high fever but I did not think much of it. I thought in my mind it would go away. Suddenly I began to feel the crisis coming up, even though I did not want anyone to know what was wrong with me, I could not hide the pain for long. It became excruciating, my Mother came into the room where I was sitting and noticed that there was something wrong. I was praying fervently that the crisis and fever would leave me but it never subsided. I was becoming delirious and shivering. Luckily, I had two uncles on board who were Doctors. They came to my rescue and bombarded me with drugs which calmed me down and made me fall into a deep slumber. I woke up with sharp pain and felt like pulling out my hair. That is something I never want to experience again in my life. I began to sing praises to God in my heart and murmuring songs. I never thought I would survive.

After a few days, we headed back to Lagos. By now the pain had subsided and I was very weak and jaundiced. The second day after arriving in Lagos, one of my uncles came to visit me at home. On seeing me, he exclaimed what! My uncle turned around to my Mother and told her 'To the hospital now'. I had to get dressed quickly with the help of my Mother. As I got to the hospital, I was transfused immediately, the jaundice had taken over my body and I was very anaemic. I spent nearly two weeks in the hospital. When I felt better, I walked around the vicinity of the hospital near the Lagoon. It was beautiful. I appreciated nature, the air was clean and fresh; for the first time in weeks I was alive!

Sickle cell is not the killer, it is the damage it does to the body, the organs do not get enough oxygen to go around the body. This causes a lot of infections that weakens the body; sometimes the organs shut down and most of the time this is what kills the sufferers.

As I survived this, I was thankful to God for seeing another era. I was alright for a month, but later I found out I was rejecting the blood I was given. I started having a crisis every month during my menstrual cycle and it lasted for three days. This went on for nearly three months or so. It left me weak each month and made me dread that period of the month. I used to go back to the hospital but there was nothing they could do but give me painkillers.

Looking over those years, I thought there was not much for me. Questions began to run through my mind, Am I going to die? Was I going to be of use to anyone? Would I get married and if I do, how would I cope? It was always one question after the other. But there was no answer to the questions for me. Therefore, I would sit and begin to ask God, what exactly was I created for, if I was of any use. It however, occurred to me that according to the Bible everyone created by God was created for a purpose. I did not know this then but deep down in my mind I knew there was something somewhere. I summoned up courage and began reframing my mind set. I was good at Arts and was quite creative. I was just a little over 21 years old then. I remember once that my father wanted to open a shop for my Mother. He called me to design a logo for the shop. I designed it beautifully. The logo was eventually used for my Mother's business.

After the age of 21, I began to withdraw and felt rejected because of this terrible illness which was no fault of mine. The illness no doubt left a dent in my life. Unfortunately, people forgot about my beauty (inner and outward) and concentrated on the dent. I felt marginalised and rejected. It was unbearable. I would describe my life then as an old book left on the shelf and read occasionally. On this premise, let me offer a word of advice to whoever is reading this book; ***Never let anyone silence or disrupt you from your desire or goals in life, Remember God gave us all a voice, shout it up on top of the roof and let everyone know about it. Shine your light, no matter how dim your light is, let it shine. The good Lord, no doubt will brighten your light. Be bold, be strong, for your Lord and God is with you.***

I got to a stage in life when I began questioning God, why me? Nothing made sense again as I began to sink into depression and low self-esteem. I felt marginalised especially when my siblings were treated nicely. Amongst us all, I was the only one who suffered from sickle cell in the family. My disease felt strange to others. My mother tried her best in every way to help, she was attending one prayer meeting after the other. She attended many for my sake with no results at the time as the pain constantly increased. I felt so lonely at the time as no one felt what I felt. I often summoned up courage when the pain got too bad and spent most times praying even though my understanding of God was limited. I wished God could heal people with the help of medicine and nature, then one way or another should work for me.

I was crying and praying one morning and kept asking God if he created me because I began to get fed up with life. It seemed as if I was going round in a circle. Life became unbearable at that stage. As I pondered over my situation God then dropped a passage in the Bible into my heart **(John 9: 1-39)**:

1 Now as Jesus passed by, He saw a man who was blind from birth. 2 And His disciples asked Him, saying, "Rabbi, who sinned, this man or his parents, that he was born blind?" 3 Jesus answered, "Neither this man nor his parents sinned, but that the works of God should be revealed in him. 4 I must work the works of Him who sent Me while it is day; the night is coming when no one can work. 5 As long as I am in the world, I am the light of the world." 6 When He had said these things, He spat on the ground and made clay with the saliva; and He anointed the eyes of the blind man with the clay. 7 And He said to him, "Go, wash in the pool of Siloam" (which is translated, Sent). So he went and washed, and came back seeing. 8 Therefore the neighbors and those who previously had seen that he was blind said, "Is not this he who sat and begged?" 9 Some said, "This is he." Others said, "He is like him." He said, "I am he." 10 Therefore they said to him, "How were your eyes opened?" 11 He answered and said, "A Man called Jesus made clay and anointed my eyes and said to me, 'Go to the pool of Siloam and wash.' So I went and washed, and I received sight." 12 Then they said to him, "Where is He?" He said, "I do not know." 13 They brought him who formerly was blind to the Pharisees. 14 Now it was a Sabbath when Jesus made the clay and opened his eyes. 15 Then the Pharisees also asked him again how he had received his sight. He said to them, "He put clay on my eyes, and I washed, and I see." 16 Therefore some of the Pharisees said, "This Man is not from God, because He does not keep the Sabbath." Others said, "How can a man who is a sinner do such signs?" And there was a division among them. 17 They said to the blind man again, "What do you say about Him because He opened your eyes?" He said, "He is a prophet." 18 But the Jews did not believe concerning him, that he had been blind and received his sight, until they called the parents of him who had received his sight. 19 And they asked them, saying, "Is this your son, who you say was born blind? How then does he now see?" 20 His parents answered them and said, "We know that this is our son, and that he was born blind; 21 but by what means he now sees we do not know, or who opened his eyes we do not know. He is of age; ask him. He will speak for himself." 22 His parents said these things because they feared the Jews, for the Jews had agreed already that if anyone confessed that He was Christ, he would be put out of the synagogue. 23 Therefore his parents said, "He is of age; ask him." 24 So they again called the man who was blind, and said to him, "Give God the glory! We know that this Man is a sinner." 25 He answered and said, "Whether He is a sinner or not I do not know. One thing I know: that though I was blind, now I see." 26 Then they said to him again, "What did He do to you? How did He open your eyes?" 27 He answered them, "I told you already, and you did not listen. Why do you want to hear it again? Do you also want to become His disciples?" 28 Then they reviled him and said, "You are His disciple, but we are Moses' disciples. 29 We know that God spoke to Moses; as for this fellow, we do not know where He is from."

30 The man answered and said to them, "Why, this is a marvelous thing, that you do not know where He is from; yet He has opened my eyes! 31 Now we know that God does not hear sinners; but if anyone is a worshiper of God and does His will, He hears him. 32 Since the world began it has been unheard of that anyone opened the eyes of one who was born blind. 33 If this Man were not from God, He could do nothing." 34 They answered and said to him, "You were completely born in sins, and are you teaching us?" And they cast him out. 35 Jesus heard that they had cast him out; and when He had found him, He said to him, "Do you believe in the Son of God?" 36 He answered and said, "Who is He, Lord, that I may believe in Him?" 37 And Jesus said to him, "You have both seen Him and it is He who is talking with you." 38 Then he said, "Lord, I believe!" And he worshiped Him. 39 And Jesus said, "For judgment I have come into this world, that those who do not see may see, and that those who see may be made blind.".

As I read this, a light switched on inside me and I was amazed! What a message. This brought a lot of encouragement and it answered a lot of questions that I had been asking. Life continued as I held on to this Bible passage, which was at the back of my mind. This was the year I believed more in God, it encouraged me to pray more. I continued in my life's journey. Whilst the condition got better a bit, I suffered occasional crises.

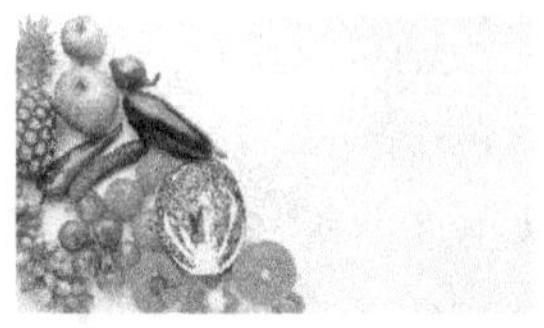

Chapter 3

The Experience of a Family Life

This is another experience of life entirely. Never jump into marriage because you want to escape problems going on in your father's house. It is wise to stop and think, make sure of where you are going, that the person you want to marry loves you for who you are and both of you can work things out simultaneously. It takes the grace of God especially for those with sickle cell disease, to live a peaceful family life.

I got married when I was 25 years old, on the 6th of Dec 1977, my marriage was a quiet one. I was happy because I was going into a new world that I had never experienced before but willing to take the risk. As my mother used to say:

"There is a price to pay for everything you do in life".

Two weeks after I married, my husband travelled to Yugoslavia, as he received a scholarship for a course in navigation. We both agreed that I would travel to the United Kingdom where he will later join me. I lived briefly with my uncle and later found a suitable accommodation for myself. At the time, I enrolled in a short course in Business studies. I suffered a few crises at the time but I found that the health system in the United Kingdom was much better than that of Nigeria. There were various accessible treatments for every illness or infection that I had. After two years of being apart from my husband, he joined me in United Kingdom. This was a new phase of my life but I was willing to forge forward and make life work for me.

At this point I never knew I could live this long let alone get pregnant. In 1980 I was expecting my first son. Everyone had given up on me, **"Que**

sera... sera; whatever would be would be" was now my new song. You know what, I was determined to do something with my life. I reflected on where I was coming from which no longer mattered and to focus on where I was going in life. I remembered the Bible Verse God gave me which in addition inspired me to move on. *(John 9:1 – 39)*

My first pregnancy was a great experience. I have petite stature and look very young for my age and pregnancy. At a point during my pregnancy, I began to struggle with my health. I kept on having crises on and off. This made me stay in hospital most of the time with no clue of what to do but mother nature thought me in no time. I began to have infections in my amniotic fluid; this got me a bit worried but I knew I was in good hands; I was under a skilled consultant of obstetrics. I believed that God was watching over me and I had gone through the worst, even passed the stage where I was supposed to die. I was only concerned about the pregnancy.

My mother flew in from Nigeria to support me. As aforementioned, I had a few sickle cell crises through my pregnancy. The worst one was a day before I went into labour. I was admitted because of my frequent false labour and was kept in hospital in order to be monitored. After a few days, a lady was brought into the ward; she had an asthma attack, she was wheezing a lot and it began to affect me, she was in so much pain I could feel it where I was. After a while she became calm from the medication she was administered. But this had affected me in a way suddenly I went into crisis and could not breath at all. It was as if my lungs were compressed, I gasped for air. I had never experienced that sort of pain before. I was given some medication to calm me down, soon after, my water broke, even though I was given medication to stop contractions thirty minutes earlier. The labour started gradually but midway things were interrupted by the doctors.

They noticed that as the contractions came the baby's heart beat dipped, there was panic in the room, this resulted in a caesarean section, to save my life and the baby's which was 37 weeks old. Although he was very strong but small, they could not keep him in the incubator for one day as he kept on pulling out the tubes put on him. As for me, after the caesarean; I had pneumonia and had to be treated for this.

I remember that during my pregnancy my mother kept on saying I should eat well. I ate a lot of vegetables and fruits; like beetroot, spinach, beans, cassava and took a lot of folic acid supplement in addition to the one I got from the food I ate. Water was also very important. I noticed nutrition helped a lot during my pregnancy because my son though was small, he was very healthy and strong. After a week and a half, we were discharged, my mother came to stay with me to help look after the baby. After about six month I decided to take up a two-year foot-wear manufacturing course. So that by the time I started the course, my son would be about one-year-old and he could start a nursery school. By the time I finished the second year of the course I was pregnant with my second son.

That was joy on its own as I began healthy eating again though this time I went on an eating spree. I managed to finish my course and passed with a good grade. I was filled with joy because I knew I was going somewhere. My eating habits had improved a lot and I thought I was doing well, only to be told six months into my pregnancy that my child was not growing as well as he should. This was a blow to me; I was told that the only thing that would solve this was if I had transfusions every two weeks. I thought 'okay' here we go again. I hated blood transfusions for reasons I cannot explain but I would do anything to give birth to a healthy baby. So, I had to go along with the treatment with no alternative choice. At this stage, my husband was confused as to what decision to make. I had to build confidence in him as he began to panic. I was already given a delivery date and I began to pray. I was a bit frightened of all these backs and forth. My second son was also born by caesarean section, because of the sickle cell and my petite stature. After the birth, I had to pray more than ever before for the pains to stop and I thank God that His promise to preserve my life was in full force. Both deliveries were a miracle of God.

A day after the surgery, the consultant came to see me and the baby, and he looked at me and looked at the baby in the cot twice and shook his head. When I asked why he did that, he said he had a difficult time birthing him; although he was breech, he had stuck his head into the lower part of my womb, and he had to twist and turn him before he could get him out. I stayed in the hospital for a while, and this was because there was a bit of complication concerning my wounds healing, they wanted to make sure everything was fine before we left. We finally got home and settled down, my mother was with me again and I thanked God for that.

At the back of my mind, I never thought I could succeed in life but I always had a feeling I would live long enough to take care of my children because my husband was always away from home. I had to cope by myself and I am sure there are others like me. I kept on telling myself **'I am fearfully and wonderfully made no matter what, I would make it in life'**. This helped me greatly, it put my mind at rest for there was a greater one than me who was going to turn my life around and that is my God who created me.

As life continues, it was not an easy journey because after my second son I became very ill. As one who suffers from sickle cell, I needed more than enough energy to cope with two children, functioning as a mother and wife at the same time. There was a crisis after three months of giving birth to my second son my husband was around with his help things were not too bad. Apart from that I began having problems digesting my food. After visiting my doctor, he sent me for some tests and they found out that I had gallstones. But they could not operate immediately because I had a caesarean section three months earlier, so I had to wait for six months. The pain was excruciating.

After six months, I had to prepare for the surgery. I was given blood transfusion a week before the surgery as I await the surgery with fear because of the pain, thought of my children and many other things. But I had to trust God with my children and my life; faced with mixed feelings, the loneliness of my childhood returned in full force, I was panicking so much I could not think straight. The surgery was performed and I was brought back to the ward in the evening. When I woke up it seemed as if I was tied down, I was so uncomfortable, I began to feel dizzy everything began to happen at once. The nurse came to take my temperature but it did not read, so she tried another thermometer. The same thing happened, at this point my body was getting cold and I could find myself slipping away. I could hear her say 'call the doctor emergency'! The only thing I could notice was that there were many of them around me and I was wrapped in foil. When I opened my eyes, I was in intensive care with all wires and instruments attached to me. I thought not again! I promised to give thanks to God if I came out of this situation. I spent a week in intensive care and another two weeks in the ward before I was discharged. My children had been taken to foster parents because my husband could not cope as he was in great distress.

Getting back home, I found it difficult to settle down as it looked like a new world to me. I also noticed that I began having one infection after the other. I found out that **those with sickle cell do not die of the sickle cell problems but infections** and this should be noted. I was given one antibiotic after another; my system was run down completely. So, I start looking for supplements to boost my immune system and change my diet to healthy eating. I found out that this helped a lot and my health began to improve again. I, therefore implore those suffering with sickle cell to ensure they eat a healthy diet with good supplements and to avoid taking iron tablets. There is sufficient iron for sickle cell sufferers from eating fresh vegetables.

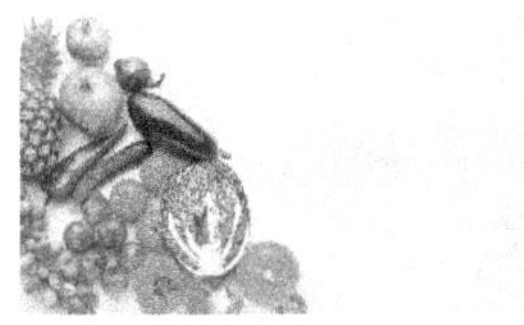

CHAPTER 4

How and When My Life Changed

After living by myself for a while a friend came to stay and spent several years with me. She was of great help as my husband was away again to study another course in marketing outside of London. My children came back home after four years and once again I became fully involved in parenthood which I enjoyed. I was so excited; it was as if I had won millions in a lottery. I began to arrange how to get the boys to attend school in London. The children finally resumed a school not too far from home and I also got a full-time job. I found it challenging taking the boys to school and back as my husband was still away studying.

In 1991 we finally moved houses, it was hectic because it took us about three months before we could settle down completely.

At this point in time I suffered sickle cell crisis quite often. My husband was called by the United Nations to Uganda and once again I was left with the children which were by now teenagers (13 and 15years old). Parenting teenagers was a bit of a challenge but I managed it successfully.

In 2006, I stepped into another era and things began to change. I had suffered several infections, asthma, chest infections... name it, it was one after the other as I was prescribed different antibiotics for every infection; I got fed up using so many antibiotics and then my immune system became erratic. I went into a crisis and was admitted into hospital. I felt rejected, depressed, and fearful for the future. At this stage I was beginning to feel weak but in all these, I had a glimpse of hope that I was more than a conqueror. Things seemingly became better as I received a lot of help and support from friends and some family members. The crisis began to subside gradually. However, going through all of the above I felt a dent in my life. The lesson I drew from this experience is that a child born with any illness is a gift from God.

Over the years, I went on to the internet searching for anything to improve my life and maximize my potential as I sensed imminent depression. One wonderful day, I stumbled upon a multi-marketing company in which I spoke to a wonderful man named John; unfortunately, John has now gone to rest in the Lord. He told me about a **Paul Barton** who could deal with my situation better. I quickly rang Paul and my victory journey began. Paul spoke to me on different occasions concerning my health, my diet and other health aids like food supplements with active ingredients containing minerals and vitamins to boost my immune system. Some of the supplements include MannaBears, Ambrotose and Phytochemicals. The supplements began to improve my health.

Paul counselled me on nutrition, I decided then to change my diet. I ate more fibers such as vegetables, fruits, nuts and seeds. My body chemistry changed as I began to look and feel very healthy. I wish I had known Paul much earlier in my life, but all the same I thank God for his mercy and grace.

Just after I started the supplements and nutrition, I was invited to a three-day Christian conference in Leeds by my sister-in-law's daughter. On the second day of the conference I fell ill and suffered a terrible crisis. I was admitted into hospital for about a week.

While at the hospital I was given a massage which helped reduce my pain. Upon discharge from hospital I was given strong painkillers to take as necessary but I had pains in my sides even after taking the painkillers so I stopped; instead I took the MannaBears. I realised that the pain went away.

After a year, I began to come off my strong pain killer, my asthma medication and other medicines. Another thing I needed to take care of was my skin. Do you know the largest organ in the body is the skin? It is therefore imperative that we take care after our skin. I suffered from eczema and no matter what I put on it, it itched a lot. I then began to look for things that were natural until I found something suitable for my skin. I remember when I was young my grandmother used coconut oil; it was called (*adiagbon*), and also my mother cooked a vegetable called (*ewuro*) which is called bitter leaf. I used to hate this because of its bitter taste. Sometimes things that are bitter are quite good for us. This is how I started the journey of nutrition, there are many other foods that I discovered that made me healthier which would be discussed subsequently.

Every individual is different and each person must find what exactly is good for them. I found out that there are common foods which everyone likes but some people are allergic to. At this point, I looked back and realised that many people had died of this disease. Some people have it more severe than others, some are deformed because of sickle cell. Food goes a long way in healing but this alone could not do the job for those with sickle cell in the interest of longevity. Thank God for some medical-scientists like **National Heart Lung and Blood Institute (NHLBI)** who are conducting expensive ongoing research to find a cure for sickle cell. Our Creator, is the main life line; according to **2 Samuel 22:2** which states that

"The Lord is my rock, my fortress, and my savior."

I therefore made a good choice to embrace my creator Yahweh in all things. He has brought me this far and done miraculous things in my life.

I realised everything that happened in my journey of life was by the grace of God, who is our loving Creator. I began to put things in place like drinking a lot of water, eating right, knowing the things that were good for my body. In the beginning, you will recall that improvement with my health was slow but as I began to build up my immune system my health improved. I was confident in coming off my medication gradually and soon learnt that the best medication lies with a balanced nutrition.

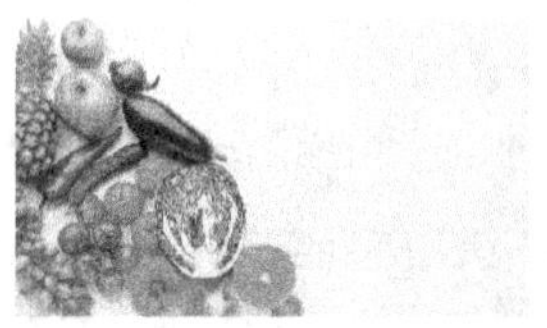

CHAPTER 5

The Power of Nutrition

Nutrition is a very important part of our lives, without it we cannot survive for long. I never knew this, until I tried eating right and using natural products on my skin. As aforementioned, you need to choose what suits you and your body will let you know if you are eating the right food. There is healing in food.

According to **Genesis 1 :28 - 29** which states:

> *"Then God blessed them and said, "Be fruitful and multiply. Fill the earth and govern it. Reign over the fish in the sea, the birds in the sky, and all the animals that scurry along the ground."*
>
> *Then God said, "look! I have given you every seed-bearing plant throughout the earth and all the fruit trees for food."*

This Bible scripture clearly reminds us that God prepared everything we needed, before he created us. He created herbs and plants for healing. At a point in time, I literally put my life in God's hands and decided to use natural things in every part of my body; internally and externally. I noticed that even when I went for my quarterly check up at the hospital the doctors were amazed. They made comments like *"you are looking very young and healthy, do not stop what you are doing"*.

Nutrition brought a lot of improvement into my life, more than I anticipated. I developed a habit of healthy eating which I still maintain to date. I presently understand how nutrition works and how it changed my DNA including my life.

According to an article by the Genetics home reference DNA or deoxyribonucleic acid which is the hereditary material in humans and almost all other organisms; nearly every cell in a person's body has the same DNA. Your DNA is what makes you uniquely you. I was amazed when I read about this in nutritional courses. Our body goes through wear and tear every day but we do not realise it. There is so much going on in our body every day, for instance when we are born the homeostasis in our body is often balanced, as we begin to grow we tend to notice what works best for our body.

It took nearly two years before I could see the effect of nutrition and supplements on my body. In fact, I never knew I could ever get better, but Paul kept on encouraging me to continue the regime of balanced nutrition and good supplements.

Apart from nutrition, water is also very important. Water helps to dilute the blood. Lack of water may cause dehydration which is a major problem that sickle cell sufferers face. I realised that beetroot is also very good for those with sickle cell; it helps with the blood and also good for maintaining the blood pressure.

Nutrition on its own can do a lot for the body and make it very healthy. Nutrition is basically *how food works*. I discovered that those suffering from sickle cell disease cannot take anything with iron in it especially if it is a pharmaceutical drug. Our body could easily digest food like vegetables which contain folic acid and iron in moderation. However, due to my condition I take food supplements, the reason being that my body needs a bit more than ordinary food and I normally would take tablets made out of natural ingredients like herbs or organic food.

My Model of Nourishing Food - *(Devised by myself)*

No	Food Sources	Nutrients	Benefits
1	Bananas	Vit B6, Potassium	Strengthens bones and teeth, promotes healthy muscles,

			protein digestion & brain function
2	Strawberries	Vit B5, C, manganese	Combats cancer, boost memory, calms stress, protects your heart
3	Sweet Potatoes	Vit A, B1, E	Good for the strengthening of bones and eyes
4	Broccoli	Vit B2, A, K	Controls blood pressure, needed to repair and maintain healthy skin
5	Beetroot	Rich in folic acid, Vit c, potassium, calcium, iron, manganese	Good for high blood pressure
6	Ugwu (fluted pumpkin leaf)	Rich in all vitamin B's and folic acid	Good for the blood and body also
7	Bitter leaf (ewuro)	Rich in folic acid and natural iron	Good for the circulation, hemoglobin a n d blood
8	Agbalumo(African star apple) Chrysophyllum Albidum	Vit C, Contains Phytochemicals such as Tannins, flavonoids, proteins terpenoids, carbohydrates and resins.	It contains more vitamin c than oranges. It lowers blood pressure and cholesterol. It can be useful in preventing and treating heart disease
9	Orin Ata (Zanthoxylum zanthoxyloides)	Sodium, Potassium, Carbohydrate, Protein, Calcium, Iron, Magnesium, Zinc and Crude Fat	It is used for the management of sickle cell aneamia It has anti-convulsant, anti-sickling, anaesthetic, anti-bacterial, anti-hypertensive and anti-inflammatory properties. It has a lot of phytochemicals
10	Ogi baba: guinea corn orSorghum spp	Magnesium, Zinc, calcium, sodium, folic acid and vitamin C	Its very important for anyone who wants maintain a healthy nervous system. This food meets the body's requirement for magnesium and zinc
11	Wonder kola (Buchholzia coriacea)	Amino acids, fatty acids, mineral such as cations (calcium, magnesium,	Has medicinal properties; used to help the nervous system,

		sodium and potassium), phosphorus, trace metals (copper, zinc, manganese, cobalt and nickel)	fibroids, diabetes, asthma and so on
12	Scent leaves: Efirin	Contains anti-fungal properties and eugenol	Can be infused as a remedy for stomach disorder such as gastroenteritis, diarrhea, cholera, chronic dysentery and vomiting. The essential oil of scent leaf has antibacterial properties, anti-fungal and Antiseptic. Used for preventing and treating malaria, catarrh, cough and fever.

Fig. 1

(i)   *(9 amazing facts you do not know about agbalumo (African star apple) by Busola Ojumu June 2nd 2016 categories, fact, health)*

(ii)   *punchng.com› nigerias-chewing-sticks-fagara zanthoxyloides*

(iii)   *13 Hidden Health Benefits of Ejinrin Leaves for Medicinal Diseases - DrHealthBenefits.com*

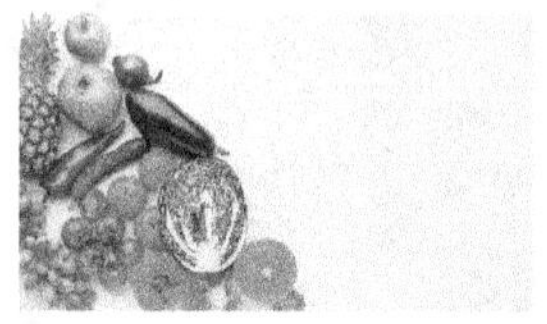

CHAPTER 6

Benefits of My Life Style Change

My golden lessons were from good nutrition and they were of great benefits. Food like carrots, quinoa, legumes, nuts and seeds etc. played a significant role in my nutritional table.

In addition to healthy eating, physical and mental changes could be seen aside from the effects of medication given at the hospital. It is routine that those with sickle cells were not given more than folic acid but my body needed more; I needed a lot of vitamins and supplements. Even people who are healthy still look for nutrients from food and supplements to make them better.

Evidently I began to look better, healthier, more alert and sharp in my thinking. I had less of a crisis with no infections at all. I believe that if I can get to this stage of my life of benefiting from nutrition and supplements, anyone can have a healthy life. Even if you have a chronic condition, it would help to start by using nutrition and its benefits to improve your body and in the long run you would appreciate the turn around to a better you.

It took a while but I conquered and never want to go back to what I was before. Improving my nutrition has been of great benefit for me. I remember there was a lady; a friend of a friend who had cancer. I am not sure what type of cancer she had but she did not go for chemotherapy and she wanted to try the options of curing her cancer with nutrition and supplements. She still lives today and she is cancer free. Although there is no cure for sickle cell, I believe one could live a pain free life. Nutrition is a process which I decided to embark on and I have never regretted it, in fact it improved my life a lot. In all this, I thank God for creating the wonderful nutritious vegetables, fruits and nuts that keep body and soul together.

Being here today is by the grace of God and sticking with what I think has been good for me, it's a pleasure to offer what I have got and done for others so that they may benefit from it too. As a wife and as a mother I incorporated these nutrients into the life of my children and family. It has paid off very well and given them a good foundation of health, and I advise all mothers to do the same.

CONCLUSION

In conclusion, I realized that if I had not taken drastic measures, I would still be perpetually in pain as doctor's advice did not yield much. And my faith in God gave me enormous victory from suffering.

After a while, with the comments of other people and my doctors, I realized I was on the right path so I continued. Not that I ignored the advice of doctors or medical professionals, I listened to their advice but it did not work so I chose an alternative way out which was to add good nutrition to my daily life and living.

Everyone looks at nutrition from a different perspective. Healthy nutrition has been tested and due to its efficacy, my advice would be for people to jump on the bandwagon and let us juggle it together. Although I went through a process, it took me where I wanted to be precisely; a place of good health. Not that there are no illnesses while using a healthy nutrition diet but they are always manageable and I recover from them very quickly.

In the beginning, it was a rough and lonely journey but I decided that I was going to get through it. I have started my journey into nature's wholeness, it's a journey of a lifetime and it continues. **You are what you eat**. We are all running a race in life and it is the survival of the fittest but one thing I have realised and come to understand is that it's only the battle that you fight that you win by God's grace.

Join in the journey of nutrition, discover the advantages and benefits it would bring to your life.

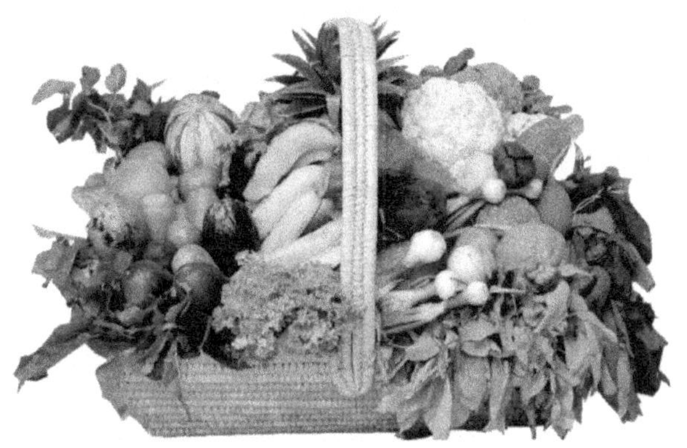

Nutritious Basket

ART
OF
LIVING
HEALTHY

FOREWORD

I've known Ruth for over 15 years and in that time she's repeatedly shown herself to be an avid learner. Given that she has full blown Sickle Cell and wasn't expected to live into her teenage years, the fact that she is still with us today suggests that she's doing something right. In fact, Ruth is a great example of 'living life to the fullest'.

There are three things that characterize Ruth; her faith, her family and her health. She manages to prioritise all three and she is an example to all around her.

Ruth's health has always been fragile and her fortitude and ability to push through very difficult circumstances is remarkable. She has an enquiring mind and is open to new concepts in terms of her health. She has even experimented with her own diet to get results that simply confound 'normal' thinking and most of all she is someone who speaks 'truth and life' to all she meets.

I'm very fortunate to count Ruth as a friend and in her own quiet way she has taught me much over the years we have known each other. Prayer is central to Ruth's very existence and if she says she is praying for you rest assured she is doing so.

In closing I'd say that Ruth is a Champion of the less fortunate and this book is a small part of that attitude working out in her day to day life.

Paul Barton

INTRODUCTION

This book has come into being because of my past challenges with ill-health over the years. This brought me to the realisation that without proper food and hydration the body does not have the capacity to survive for a long period of time and the immune system becomes weak. This serves as a catalyst and an invitation to many illnesses and infections. Therefore, proper nutrition becomes essential.

To a believer in God, our body is the Temple of God. He has provided for our needs concerning all types of food and if we adhere to this belief our body will function correctly, as it was created to be. It was through my journey in nutrition and implementing various sources of food that I regained my health. We can all live healthy and adventurous lives through good nutrition.

Nutrition is the process of providing or obtaining the necessary food for health and growth. These same principles apply to those whose bodies are plagued with disease or want to lose weight or address any ill- health concerns. Living a healthy life that is free from disease is possible.

The body is one unique creation of God that it is made up of so many parts and God has put each part just where he wants it as they all work simultaneously together as a whole. The human body communicates on all levels and the organs are all linked to one another; internally the body has a reasonably stable environment and if this is destabilized for one reason or the other, the body does not work properly. The only way to bring it back to stability is to feed it with nutrients and fluid to balance it again.

Our bodies are wonderfully and fearfully made by God. According to **Genesis 1: 29-30:**

> *"God said, "I give you every seed-bearing plant on the face of the whole earth and every tree that has fruit with seed in it. They will be yours for food. And to all the beasts of the earth and all the birds in the sky and all the creatures*

that move along the ground—everything that has the breath of life in it—I give every green plant for food." And it was so. **(NIV)**

God has created all things for our survival and has put different types of food in place for us like herbs, plants, fruits, vegetables, etc. that bring the body back to good health. For instance, in our cars, when we fill them with petrol, water, engine oil and other essential requirements needed for them to run, they will work efficiently. But if diesel is put in a car that uses petrol, that could potentially damage the engine and ultimately destroy the car. The human body is far more sophisticated than cars, it does require the appropriate nutrients to function properly as it was created to. The word of God is our manual for life, it helps us know our God more intimately. Proper nutrition is how to care for our bodies.

We need to feed our body with healthy food and make every effort not to neglect it. Food, sleep, exercise and water are needed for the perfect functioning of the body. God created plants, herbs and animals. Adam named them all, each is embedded with a code.

We are created in the image of God and we have his DNA in us. Deoxyribonucleic (DNA) this stands for the key foundation on which the structure of life is built. The seeds of these plants are sown into the ground to germinate and grow into plants; in other words, animals reproduce of their own kind. When we are confronted with disease or illness and we eat a particular plant or herb or a combination of both, the codes in the plants align with the codes created in us by God and this heals the body and makes it whole again.

In the bible **Psalm 139:13-16** says:

> *"You formed my innermost being, shaping my delicate inside and wove them all together in my mother's womb----"*

(Passion Bible)

For example, if a washing machine made by either Sony or Samsung breaks down, repair is required with the specific components produced to make the device operate again. If a part meant for a Sony electrical device is fitted into a Samsung device, it would not work. But if the correct and appropriate parts are fitted into the washing machine it would function effectively.

Science is phenomenal and appreciable and has brought about modern medicine but not without side effects. God has created everything with a solution and with no side effects. For instance, God created some plants to work perfectly in healing the human body. The human body recognizes the code in plants, herbs, vegetables and makes use of them as needed, therefore we need to go back to the origin of God's plan for a wholesome body.

Science is wonderful in supporting some of God's plans. A lot has been discovered through science. Medications recommended by renowned pharmacologists have used natural food and herbs as evidence of a good healing process.

Therefore, using natural food could serve as a good aid in all healing processes. Modern science has combined a lot of chemicals with natural food in speeding up the process of healing in the human body. However, complementary medicine has considered natural food as the best aid for healing.

The purpose of this book on nutrition is to bring us back to healthy eating so we can live healthily because health is wealth. There are so many factors that can cause the body to become under-nourished such as our environment, diseases, lack of eating nutritious food and not drinking enough water. The body is made up of about 70% of water. When it becomes dehydrated this causes the body numerous problems. Later in the book, there will be discussions of the different types of illnesses, what you can eat to keep the body healthy and how the body can be restored to its original state through proper nutrition, the use of vitamins, minerals and supplements, as well as through exercise and sleep which are both equally important.

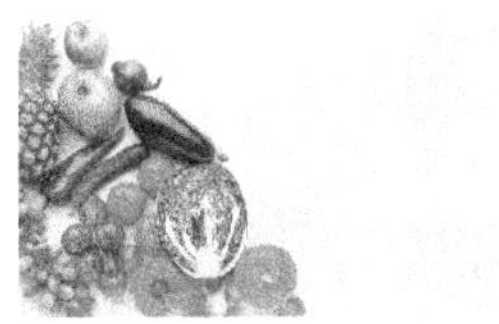

Nutrition

7.1 What is nutrition?

A good definition of nutrition was sighted in a website: Encyclopedia.com/science and technology

Whereby nutrition is defined as the combined process involved in eating and the utilizing of food substances, which are then used for the vital functioning of all parts of the body.

The body uses the food consumed for strength, growth, repair and maintenance.

The body needs about six nutrients from food to make it healthy. These are **Carbohydrates, Protein, Fat, Fibre, Vitamins, Minerals and Water**. Water is the most important of all. Although all other nutrients have their place in our diet. Nutrition is the life-line of human beings and without it the body will not function properly.

In my view, God created everything perfectly and every nutrient in each vegetable, fruit, and nut has its importance in the body. They strengthen the immune system, the digestive system and all other systems. The human body is inter-woven and all systems work harmoniously to make it whole. It is often said that *'we are what we eat.'*

7.2 The Benefits of Nutrition

There are many benefits of nutrition, and if we eat healthy, all parts of the body would benefit from the consumption. As earlier stated, every person should endeavour to eat a balanced diet as this helps all the systems of the body to function harmoniously not just for a moment but for a lifetime. This makes a healthy lifestyle, whereby the immune system maintains its strength and fights off many diseases, if not all.

In addition; a *Sharecare* article states that the benefits of good nutrition are multiple. Besides helping you maintain a healthy weight, good nutrition is also essential for the body and all its systems to function optimally for a lifetime. In fact, the benefits of good nutrition can be found in physical and mental health because a healthy diet provides energy, promotes good sleep and gives the body what it needs to stay healthy. When you consider the benefits of good nutrition, it's easier to eat healthy.

Sharecare- www.sharecare.com/health/nutrition-diet/articles

http://www.medicalonline.com.au/medical/nutrition/benefits-of-good-nutrition.htm

7.3   Advantages of Nutrition

Nutrition can help control weight, maintain a healthy heart and keep a good digestive system. Eating healthily and following a balanced diet would keep away those diseases that damage our health system.

Neal yard How Food works DK pg 12, 13

Neal's yard recommends that it is most desirable to eat things like vegetables, fruits, nuts, seeds and grains, to also include carbohydrates, protein and good fats. Truly the vegetable kingdom contains our best medicine.

Fruit and vegetables provide the principal alkaline minerals, like calcium, potassium and magnesium. They are full of phytonutrients with many health promoting attributes including antioxidants, anticancer and auto-inflammatory properties. It is therefore advisable that organic produce should be bought, to preserve its nutritional value.

7.4   Malnutrition

A further study compiled by *Neal yard* explains that Malnutrition results from a diet that does not contain the appropriate amount of nutrients. The lack of carbohydrates and proteins can lead to major development and growth problems. Deficiency in certain vitamins and minerals can cause specific illnesses for example, a lack of iron in some cases may lead to anaemia.

Over nutrition however, occurs when an oversupply of nutrients causes health problems such as obesity caused by a high- calorie diet.

Neal's study also describes Cholesterol as a waxy fatlike substance found in every cell of our bodies. There are good and bad cholesterol levels, the good is made by the liver and it is vital for normal body function. Bad cholesterol is what is called high cholesterol; if an excess of this builds up in the blood, it causes problems such as heart disease and may affect the bones, teeth, and every other part of the body.

Questions:

1. How would you rate your diet?
2. Do you eat healthily or do you grab anything accessible and available?

3. Would you classify yourself overweight or the right size for your height

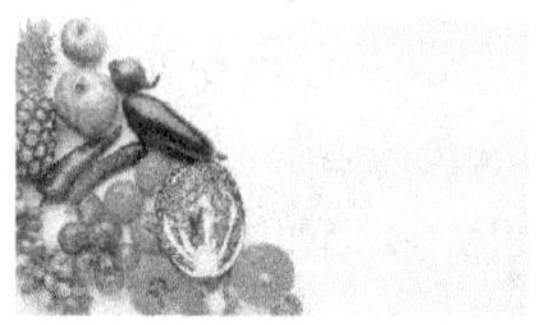

CHAPTER 8

The Nutrients in Food

Do you know God created all living things perfectly? In the beginning God made everything good. He specified in the bible what good foods to eat. **(Genesis 1:29-30),** foods that heal, like herbs, fish, meat etc. It is the joy of the Lord to see us all healthy because we are the temple of the creator- God.

There are various nutrients in food, which enable the body to grow and provide energy. Each fruit and vegetable has its specific nutrients including different minerals and vitamins required for the organs, cells, muscles and the blood. Each component provides its own strength for the immune system as well as other systems.

A learning program devised by *Byjus*, gave a detailed explanation on types of organs in a human body:

- The human body is composed of *trillion cells* which are considered as the fundamental unit of life.
- The group of *similar cells* with similar functions forms a *tissue*.
- These *tissues* combine together to form *organ systems* which finally give rise to an *individual*.

www.byjus.com

Altogether, there are seventy-eight main organs within the human body. These organs work in coordination to give rise to several organ systems. Among these 78 organs, five organs are considered as vital for survival. These include the **Heart, Brain, Kidneys, Liver and Lungs**. If any of these five organs stop functioning even for a few seconds, death will result if there is any medical intervention. Therefore, it is always advisable that we keep our system healthy, maintain a balanced diet, adequate sleep, regular physical activities and focus on healthy lifestyle changes. In most cases, when a system or the body malfunctions, these nourishing foods can correct and re-position the body bringing it back into wholeness.

The seven nutrients which the body requires are namely carbohydrates, fibre, proteins, fat, vitamins, minerals and water being most important. Each has specific nutrients in them performing specific tasks and functions in the system of the body. As you progress on this journey of exploration, you will discover these nutrients and their importance.

8.1   Carbohydrates

Carbohydrates are a form of energy. They are sourced from sugars, starch, fibres from fruits, vegetables, grains and milk products. Carbohydrates contain hydrogen, carbon and oxygen atoms. They are actually a life-line to the body as water is to a camel. There are two types of carbohydrates: *simple carbohydrates* and *complex carbohydrates*:

- ➢ Simple carbohydrates are easily digested and found in refined foods like white bread, rice, cakes and pasta. Simple carbohydrates, therefore have the capacity to enable weight gain if eaten in unguarded proportions. They also enable one to obtain a quick rush of energy.

- ➢ Complex carbohydrates are found in foods like whole-grain bread, beans, chickpeas and cereals. They are slow-releasing energy foods which are broken down over a longer period of time. These are healthy carbohydrates, high-fibre and a key part of a nutritious and healthy diet.

8.2   Proteins

Proteins are one of the vital nutrients that the body requires. They are broken down by the body, into building blocks and are used to make new proteins as well as other complex molecules. Although proteins can serve as an energy source, their main function is creation, growth and the repair of the tissues in the body.

In addition, proteins are complex molecules made up of many amino-acids connected in a chain. Amino acids are small molecules made from carbon, hydrogen, oxygen and nitrogen. There are 21 types in the human body. Our bodies are not able to supply all the essential proteins it requires, it is therefore necessary to consume these essential amino acids from our food.

Fortunately, these types of proteins can be sourced from animal products and are called complete proteins. They can be obtained from grains like Quinoa and also from nuts and seeds. It is therefore important to understand that proteins perform necessary functions in our body. It builds up our muscles and enables vital chemical processes.

8.3   Fibre

Fibre is a component of food that cannot be broken down by the body since it is made up of substances such as cellulose, lignin and pectin, which are all resistant to the action of the digestive enzyme.

There are 2 types of fibre: soluble and insoluble. Both are important for health, digestion and disease prevention.

> ➢ The *MedlinePlus* medical encyclopaedia asserts that soluble fibre attracts water and turns to gel during digestion. This process slows digestion and softens our stool which helps avoid constipation. Soluble fibre is found in oat bran, barley, nuts, seeds, beans, lentils, peas and some fruits and vegetables. It is also found in psyllium, a common fibre supplement.

> ➢ Insoluble fibre, however, does not dissolve in water and is left intact as food moves through the gastrointestinal tract. Wholegrain foods such as wheat, brown rice, couscous, root vegetables such as

carrots, parsnips, potatoes, celery, cucumbers and curettes all contain insoluble fibre.

www.medlineplus.gov/ency/article/002458.htm

Fibres are carbohydrates composed of long chains of sugar molecules and are different from other carbohydrates because they are not easy to digest in the stomach. Many people have insufficient fibre in their diet, which is a major cause of constipation. Whole grains are a good source of fibre if the fibre-rich outer part is not removed.

Fibre is also important as it can prevent the risk of some diseases like heart disease, obesity and type 2 diabetes to mention a few. Fibre is a rich source of food for the gut flora- the good bacteria in our gut.

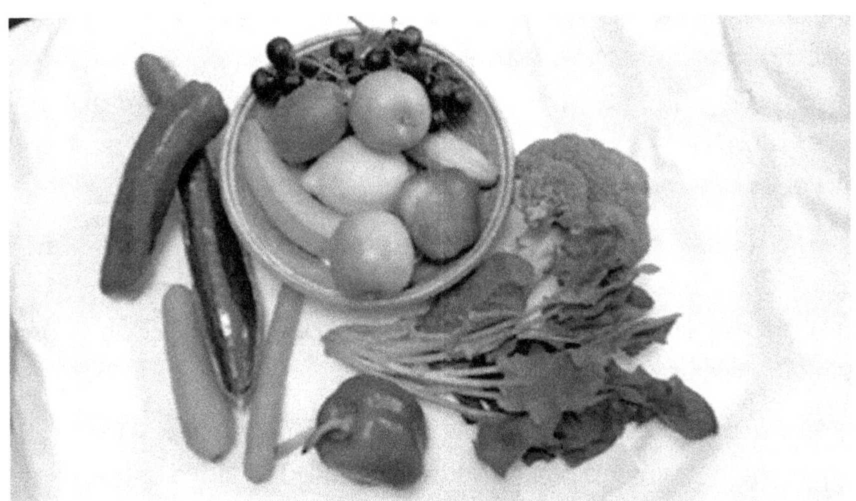

Fibre-rich foods

Our bodies are made up of a myriad of systems and each one requires certain nutrients to perform optimally and all working in harmony.

The nutrients in our food feed our body, to make new cells. It also feeds our muscles to make them strong. If we eat nourishing food, it contributes greatly to our well-being. God knew us before we were formed in our mother's wombs. He did an excellent job in creating us, giving us tools and directions on how to take maximum care of ourselves.

Our bodies respond directly to a healthy diet. This is the rationale behind correct food consumption, speedy recovery during ill health and healing process. It is our responsibility to keep our bodies healthy and in good shape. We are God's temple so we need to be healthy to enable us to carry out His work.

"By His divine power, God has given us everything we need for living a godly life.

(2 Peter 1:3 NLT)

God has given us all we need spiritually, physically with proper nutrition.

8.4   Fat

According to information sighted in *'How food works'*, Fats in specified quantities are another essential nutrient for our bodies, as they make us healthy, providing energy while storing the remainder of calories for later use. Fat has other roles it plays in the body, like forming cell membranes and making hormones.

Some fats are body friendly and essential to a healthy diet. They are foods for our brain to help keep it sharp. Fats help our cells function at optimal rates and protect our body organs by absorbing vitamins found in our diet. Therefore, we should eat healthy fats, for example nuts and seeds.

Fats are involved in constructing and repairing nervous tissues, they maintain healthy skin and nails, they are also used to make hormones that control blood pressure, the immune system, growth and blood clotting.

Only two fatty acids are essential out of all the fatty acids, this being because the body is unable to produce these; **Omega 3** and **Omega 6** fatty acids. Omega 3 fatty acid is called alpha-linoleic acid. This can be found in fish oil and fish such as salmon and mackerel. Omega 6 fatty acid is called linoleic acid. Both types of fatty acids are found in nuts and seeds. Fat makes up the third class of macronutrients together with carbohydrates and proteins.

Macronutrients are a combination of protein, carbohydrates and fat. Micronutrients are a combination of vitamins and minerals.

Other beneficial fruits and properties: -

Beetroot

Beetroot is a very good source of folic acid and it is very good for those who have sickle cell.

It contains vitamin C, rich in potassium; the leaves are rich in beta carotene, calcium and iron. The iron in beetroot is natural because it is from food therefore, it is safe to consume in moderation. It helps with anaemia and also with our blood count; it boosts the energy in the body also. Beetroot stimulates the immune system and it could be eaten raw or cooked but it is best eaten raw in salads. Beetroot is good for those who have high blood pressure. Juicing is also a very good practice to incorporate into our food regime for nutrient maximization.

Avocado Pear

According to *ehealthzine* avocados are considered a nutrient dense fruit as they are loaded with a huge variety of vitamins and minerals. It is also high in fibre and contains phytochemical like beta-sitosterol, glutathione, lutein and zeaxanthin. Moreover, avocados are one of the few fruits that contain monounsaturated fat, which is a "good" fat. It is good for the heart, and the fibre in it helps to regulate blood sugar. It also has vitamin K, E, C, vitamin B complex and potassium.

15 Health Benefits of Avocado (ehealthzine.com) by Hezy Evans | April 20, 2011

Garden Egg

Further research also revealed that garden eggs are a good source of dietary fibre as well as other minerals and vitamins such as vitamin B1, potassium, folate, manganese, magnesium, copper, Vitamin B6, niacin and other various secret nutrients.

Finelib.com

THIOCYANATE

Foods containing Thiocyanate and some Fats - in alphabetical order

African yam (note 1)	Cassava	Millet
Alfalfa sprouts	Cassava flour	Mustard
Apricot	Cauliflower	Green Onion - raw
Apricot kernels	Cherry	Peaches
Bamboo shoot	Chickpea	Plantain
Banana	Cloudberry	Plantain flour
Beetroot (raw – note 2)	Elderberry	Plums
Bitter almond	Flaxseed	Pounded yam
Broccoli	Garlic	Radish sprouts
Brussels sprouts	Grains	Raspberry
Buckwheat	Grasses	Red Clover
Buffalo berry	Kohlrabi	Rutabaga
Cabbage	Lentils	Salmonberry
Carrot	Lima bean	Sorghum
	Macadamia nuts	Strawberry
		Turnips

Table 1

According to research findings the apparent rarity of Sickle Cell in Africa was put down to a 'mysterious protective agent'. It may be possible that this 'agent' is in fact dietary Thiocyanate. A close study conducted by science directly found that as a competitive inhibitor of the sodium iodide symporter at thiocyanate level (NIS) normally found in blood, they are also known as rhodanide. Thiocyanate is one of the most important spectrophotometric reagents. I will in the future be writing a journal on thiocyanate properties and its effects with nutrition.

www.sciencedirect.com

Thiocyanate is highest in foods that are commonly eaten in Africa – African yams (see left picture) and cassava or Manioc (plus a few others). According to research findings, for many years

Thiocyanate could also account for the higher occurrence and greater severity of sickle cell in the Westernised African population, in North

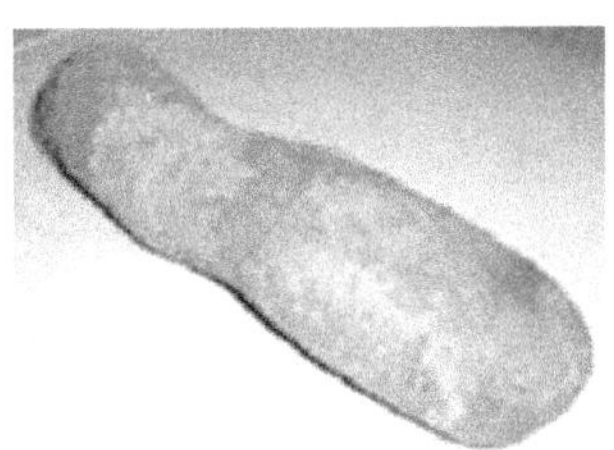

America and Europe. The African diet, without western influence, contains about 40 times more Thiocyanate than a comparable western diet. Sweet potatoes are also a good source except the ones grown in the US.

8.5   Vitamins

In view of research carried out by *Neal yard studies*; Vitamins are organic compounds and essential nutrients that human beings need. They are a group of micronutrients found in different types of vegetables and fruits which are essential for our growth, vitality and well-being.

The body produces some of these and others obtainable from the food we eat.

They also control the metabolic process, such as vitamin C and E, and act as antioxidants. We derive most of these necessary vitamins from a complete healthy diet and the rest from supplements. The body only needs minimal amounts. However, the lack of any of the above may be potentially dangerous, and may lead to different types of diseases.

Vitamins are classified according to how they dissolve in fats or water. Those that dissolve in fat are called fat- soluble vitamins which are mainly found in fatty foods such as eggs, fish, and dairy food.

How Food Works

Vitamins	Functions
A Also, known as **Beta-carotene**	Needed for vision, growth and development: foods examples, Beef liver, carrots, sweet potatoes, tomatoes, broccoli mangoes, pumpkins, apricot, papaya, Pumpkin leaf (Telfaria Occidentalis) aloe vera
B1	Helps generate energy and ensures muscles and nerves function well Food examples: Watercress, courgette, mushrooms, peas, cauliflower, tomatoes, Brussels sprouts, beans, pumpkin leaf (Telfaria occidentalis)
B2	Important for metabolism and healthy skin, eyes and nervous system Food examples: Mushrooms, asparagus, cabbage, beansprouts, strawberry, mackerel,
B3	Maintains the nervous system and brain, the cardiovascular system, the blood metabolism. Food examples: Mushroom, chicken, salmon, lamb, turkey, pumpkin leaf
B5	Important for metabolism and in the production of neurotransmitters, hormones and haemoglobin Food examples: Mushrooms, celery, strawberries, broccoli, avocados and so on
B6	Involved in nerve function, metabolism and making antibodies as well and haemoglobin Food examples: Wheat germ, watercress, bananas, red kidney beans, onions
B7	Biotin, needed for healthy bones, hair and fat metabolism Food examples: Egg yolk, soya beans, brewer's yeast
B9	Folic acid, for vital healthy infants Food examples: Spinach, sesame seeds, avocados, cashew nuts, cauliflower
B12	Promotes active metabolism and formation of red blood cells, Food examples: Oysters, eggs, cottage cheese, sardines, Turkey, aloe vera
C	An antioxidant that helps the growth and repair of various tissue throughout the body Food examples: Peppers, strawberries, lemon, oranges, melon, tomatoes, pumpkin leaves, aloe vera

D3	Aids uptake of some minerals Food examples: Herrings, mackerel, eggs, salmon. D3 offers many health benefits, it is known to help strengthen bones, muscles, it boosts immunity, increases mood aids in weight loss and improves heart function. www.verywellhealth.com written 16/10/2020
E	An antioxidant protects cell membranes, maintaining healthy skin and eyes, and strengthens the immune system. Food examples: Sunflower seeds, tuna, unrefined cold-press oil, aloe vera
K	Needed to make blood-clotting agents. Food examples: Cauliflower, cabbage, potatoes, corn oil, lettuce

Table 2

8.6 Minerals

The global healing center recommends that Minerals are required for the body to function properly. Health topics research further conducted by *Medline plus* also revealed that there are two kinds of minerals: **macro minerals and trace minerals**. A recent study of 19th Oct 2020 giving concerns of Covid 19 recommended larger amounts of macro minerals. They include calcium, phosphorus, magnesium, sodium, potassium, chloride and sulfur. We only need small amounts of trace minerals. These occur naturally in certain foods enlisted in the table below:

www.medlineplus.gov -Medline plus - study of 19th Oct 2020 giving concerns of Covid 19

www.verywellhealth.com written 16/10/2020

MINERALS	MACROMINERALS FUNCTIONS	SOURCES OF MINERALS
Calcium	Needed for blood clotting, muscle function, nerve transmission, builds up bones teeth and keeps them strong. Maintains the correct acid-alkaline balance.	Eggs, Sesame Seed, Water Melon, Tinned Sardines, Cocoyam, Stockfish, Black-Eyed Beans, Cheddar Cheese, Almonds, Corn Tortillas.

Magnesium	Play an important role in the formation of the teeth and bones. Also useful for transmitting nerves signals and heart muscles and nervous system	Wholegrain Cereals, Ginger, Cloves, Watermelon, Fresh and Dried Prawns, Pawpaw, Sorghum, Maize or Millet Pap, Okra, Almonds, Peanuts, Cashew Nuts. Garlic
Phosphorus	Useful for formation of bones and teeth, also needed to release energy in cells. It's a component of DNA and RNA, helps maintain ph of the body	Present in All Animal and Plant Protein Such as Cheese, Red Meat, Avocado, Plantain Its Present in Almost All Foods
Potassium	Mineral and a salt (sodium) to keep the balance of fluid and electrolyte in the cells. It also corrects the ph balance in the body. Helps secretion of insulin for blood sugar control to produce constant energy.	Avocado, Banana, Oranges, Nuts, Yam, Mango Tiger Nuts Almonds, Salmon, Coconut Water, Mushrooms, Molasses
Sodium	Necessary for maintaining water balance in the body as well as muscle and nerve function, to prevent dehydration. Helps move nutrients into cells.	Rock Salt, Baobab Leaves, Fermented Egusi Seeds. Olives, Shrimps, Ham, Celery, Cabbage.
Chromium	Important for regulation of blood sugar levels, improves lifespan, helps protect DNA and RNA. Essential for heart function.	Red Meat, Liver, Molasses, Seafood, Apples, Wholemeal Bread, Parsnips.
Copper	Assists in production of pigment in eyes, hair and skin, helps the body to absorb iron	Mushrooms, Oysters, Ginger, Nutmeg, Liver

MINERALS	MACROMINERALS FUNCTIONS	SOURCES OF MINERALS
Iron	Major component of the red pigment, haemoglobin in blood which carries oxygen around the body. Important for energy production	Groundnut, Cloves, Soya Beans, Sugar Cane, Guinea Fowl, Bitter Leaf

Manganese	Required for the proper functioning of enzymes	Brown Rice, Garlic Onion, Pineapple, Whole Grain Bread
Selenium	Aids adequate functioning of the immune system and thyroid gland. Antioxidant mineral: this protects cell from free radicals	Mackerel, Brazil Nuts, Lentils,
Sulphur	Promotes production of amino acids and the insulin hormone	White Seed Melon, Nuts, Meat, Seafood
Zinc	Essential for normal cell division growth and repair. Also used to maintain a health immune system	Black-Eyed Beans, Oysters, Avocado, Sesame Seeds

Table 3

Macro minerals are present at larger levels in the animal body and required in larger amounts in the diet. Aforementioned, they include calcium, chlorine, magnesium, phosphorus, potassium, sodium and sulphur.

These rich minerals are often referred to as trace minerals, meaning they are present at low levels in the body and required in smaller quantities in the animal's diet. They include chromium, cobalt, copper, fluorine, iodine, iron, manganese, molybdenum, selenium and zinc.

This section was written because it was extremely helpful when I decided to start the journey of eating a healthy diet. There were foods that I intentionally integrated into my diet which resulted in improved nutrition for my body and contributed a wealth of good to my well-being. Human beings are of varying compositions and a certain type of food may not be agreeable with one person but may be perfect for another. Also, remember to consume everything in moderation.

Balance is the key to life and too much of everything can be harmful to the body.

(i)   Neal's Yard- How food works from DK
(ii)   Global healing centre: https://www.globalhealingcenter.com/
(iii)   www.Medlineplus.gov

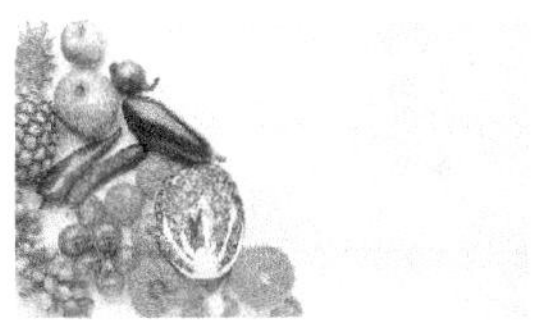

CHAPTER 9

Water

9.1 What is the importance of water?

Water is very important to the body; without it we cannot live. It is the life line of every living creature and being, from human beings to plants and animals. Water is the body's most important nutrient, it is involved in every bodily function and makes up 60- 70% of total body weight. It helps to maintain body temperature, metabolize body fat, aids in digestion, lubricates and cushions organs, transports nutrients and flushes toxins from your body.

Dr Christopher Vasey, Naturopathic Doctor in his book - ***The Water Prescription*** said

> *"Drinking sufficient quantities of water is a necessity for optimal physical functioning but it can also play a major role in the prevention and treatment of many diseases".*

Chronic fatigue, depression, eczema, rheumatism, gastric disorders, high or low blood pressure, high cholesterol, obesity and urinary infections are but a few of the many disorders that can result from not drinking enough water and which can be treated by raising our intake of this vital liquid.

9.2 The Uses and Benefits of Water

Water is a major component in completing the simplest task. It forms the base of our saliva, forms the fluids in our joints, regulates body temperature, alleviates constipation, prevents dry skin, may aid in the prevention of colon, bladder and breast cancer and regulates our appetites and metabolism. Most people often confuse hunger for food with thirst. Thirst is just one of many of the body's ways of indicating that it needs water.

There is another type of water called kangen water, it makes the body alkaline. Our brain is about 85% water so if that level drops, brain function may decrease. Our bodies are composed of water for a very important reason - to maintain good health and to keep our body fluids healthy as our body mass is composed of a higher proportion of water.

If our intake of water is high or low, the body will signal this deficiency by either absorbing more water into the cells or flushing out excess from the cells. In both cases, this is damaging. Water is important to all organs especially the brain, the eye, blood and digestive system; all the organs work in conjunction with each other.

Brain Hydration: Water is important for the brain to function, the balance between water and the substance dissolved in it is important for neurons to transmit signals effectively. In our bodies, the brain is made up of ninety-five percent water. Without proper amounts of water, our bodies become dehydrated and cannot function. Intense dehydration can lead to black outs; however, mild symptoms can include hunger, difficulties in focusing and fatigue.

Eyes: Water is a major component used in the eyes, it keeps the eyes clean and comfortable and this is done by the eyes producing tears to moisturise it.

Blood: Blood fluid is 92% water. The liquid allows oxygenated blood cells, infection fighting white cells and other vital components to flow exactly where they are needed.

Digestive system: Water aids digestion. The acidic liquid in your stomach is part water, mixes with your food and helps to digest it. The liquid in the intestines help to move the digested food along easily. When the body is well hydrated, urine is pale in colour. On the other hand, if the body is dehydrated, urine becomes dark in colour. Food passes through the large intestine and the body absorbs water from it. This leaves the stool dry and hard causing constipation.

9.3   Alkaline water

I discovered alkaline water in 2006 when I embarked on taking supplements for the first time. It was called *Kangen* water, I had never heard of it prior to that time, but since then it has been of great benefit to my body. As a sufferer of sickle cell anaemia, *Kangen* water has also enabled my body to function more efficiently, especially due to the medication and antibiotics that were prescribed. These made my body become quite acidic, thus causing a lot of problems. Acidity affects the immune system and attracts more diseases. Every person is different from the other therefore if you embark on a regimen of supplements, vitamins or food that is not agreeable to your body, take a break from using it or stop using completely.

9.3.1 What is alkaline water?

Alkalinity and acidity are both measurements on the pH scale of 1 to 14. Neutral is considered 7.0 and anything below that point is considered acidic. Alkaline water typically has a pH between 7.0 and 10.0 on the scale.

Another common name for alkaline water is ionized water. It is thought that natural spring water is the best source of alkaline water, with a pH around 8.0 to 9.0. Alkaline water also has a higher pH level than tap water. Regular tap water usually has a pH level of 6.0 to 7.0.

Natural alkaline water occurs when water travels over rocks. For instance, spring water will obtain minerals and increase in alkalinity during this process. Basically, spring water is naturally alkalized.

However, there are products called alkaline ionizers that alkalinize the water during electrolysis. It is a chemical process that separates water into more acidic or alkaline molecules. Alkaline water and water ionizers are typically found in many health foods stores or grocery stores.

9.3.2 The health benefits of alkaline water

According to *The Health Science Academy*, alkaline water helps to turn our acidic body back to an alkaline body. This is particularly good for people who consume diets that are acidic for the body, for example processed food, dairy, sugar and red meat. Other alkaline benefits are as follows:

1.   It helps to detoxify: -

Detoxification is important for removing the accumulation of harmful toxins in the body. Overload of toxins can lead to chronic fatigue, low energy, bloating, mental confusion, inflation and food sensitivities.

2.   It helps in weight loss plan: -

According to the study in the journal *Original internist (2011)*, it is beneficial in losing weight. Researchers found that obese individuals who drank 2 litres of alkaline water daily, lost an average of 12lbs over 2 months.

3.   Reduces acid reflux: -

Helps with indigestion and heartburn. It also inactivates pepsin, an enzyme that plays a role in acid reflux.

4.   Helps improve bone health: -

Alkaline water can improve bone health.

5.   Provides antioxidant benefits: -

Alkaline water is a natural antioxidant that can neutralise harmful radicals in the body.

6.   It is essential for heart health: -

Drinking alkaline water can reduce certain risk factors associated with heart disease. In a study conducted in 2011, by the *Original Internist researchers* found that alkaline water consumption for three to six months could significantly reduce blood pressure, blood sugar and cholesterol.

Natural products are lemon ginger, organic pure honey and water, also another type of water called Kegan water.

In conclusion, alkaline ionized water will help those with symptoms associated with diabetes and hypertension. Heart disease and hypertension are risk factors for diabetes. Drinking alkaline water may also help hydrate your body, improve mental clarity and boost your overall immune system.

Roddy Macdonald Founder & Managing Director of Water for Health

Dr. Christopher Vasey, Naturopathic Doctor in his book - The Water Prescription

Questions

1. How much water do you drink in a day?

2. Is sparkling water or soft drinks good for you?

3. Do you drink fizzier drinks than water?

4. What do you think about drinking alkaline water, and would you try it?

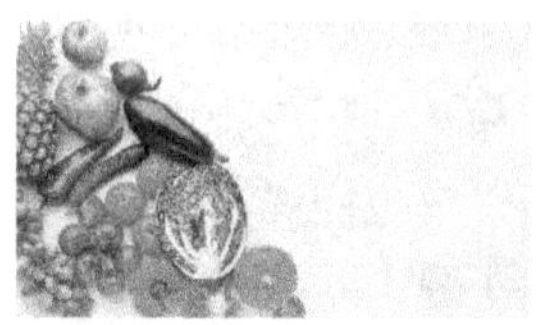

CHAPTER 10

Detoxification

According to **Laura Harris Smith**:

"I acknowledge that God has created several of our key organs to do all our detoxing for us. The liver, kidneys, skin and lungs are already excellent filters capable of handling the typical environmental contaminants that throw themselves at the body (or hide in food). Filters however, get dirty – Overtaxed, so the purpose of the physical portion of this detox is to baby your body, disinfect your filtration system and free up your organs to do their jobs better."

Smith, Laura Harris. The 30-Day Faith Detox (p. 21), Baker Publishing Group. Kindle Edition.

10.1   What is detoxification?

This is the process of eliminating poisonous or waste substances(toxins) from the body or to neutralise adverse effects.

Although our bodies detoxify naturally, excessive exposure to toxins through poor diet or lifestyle can lead to toxins accumulating faster than the body can eliminate them. An effective body detox moves waste, allowing the body to function better.

A healthy person has no reason to detox because the body has a healthy mechanism which detoxes naturally. It is only when we expose ourselves to excessive toxins through poor diet or lifestyle, that we need to detox, so the body can get rid of these toxins and manage to get back to its natural way of keeping the body safe from free radicals and toxins.

Transforming your diet and lifestyle to a more alkaline diet will result in the body naturally getting rid of toxins and excess acidity it stores. Detoxification can also aid weight loss; as excess fat is always an acid problem.

10.2   What are Toxins?

A toxin is any substance that causes harm on getting into our body. There are toxic substances all around us and they can be classified into three groups depending on their origin. The liver and kidneys, neutralise or expel excess harmful chemicals.

Internal toxins

The body is tuned to fighting impurities to keep us alive and flushes out unwanted impurities in the system, digests food, pumps blood around the body, metabolises and assimilates nutrients. What happens to all the by-products of these processes? In a perfectly healthy body, millions of cells die every day, these and other by-products need to be removed to avoid clogging the systems and this is done by the body's natural process of detoxification.

External toxins

These are toxins we are exposed to daily, such as junk food or contaminated water. Environmental pollutants could be in the form of smog, chemicals in lotions, creams, soaps used on the skin and are absorbed partially. The skin is the largest organ of the body so special care is needed to take care of it. Other toxins are side effects from pharmaceutical medicines we take, dental procedures, chemicals in household goods and even insect bites.

10.3   Toxic lifestyles

Poor lifestyles can stress the body. It reduces the ability to detoxify itself, thereby toxins accumulate.

Toxic behaviour includes lack of sleep and rest, lack of exercise, stress, poor diet and not drinking enough water.

10.4 Warning signposts of a need to detox the body

The body has a mechanism where it sends out warning signals when it needs to be detoxed. The following symptoms may appear when the body needs to be detoxed:

- Skin diseases: acne, eczema, dermatitis, hives, psoriasis, brittle nails, hair loss.
- Lungs: (respiratory problems): asthma, bronchitis, emphysema, sinusitis.
- Colon: bad breath, body odour, constipation, diarrhea, excessive flatulence, irritable bowel syndrome (IBS), gastritis, heartburn, indigestion, stomach ulcer.
- Liver: cirrhosis, jaundice, gall-bladder stones, hepatitis.
- Kidneys: kidney stones, urinary tract disorders.
- Lymphatic system: varicose veins, glandular fever, lymph nodes disease, Hodgkin's disease, elephantiasis.
- General mental health: irritability, poor memory, insomnia, chronic fatigue, headaches, migraines, depression.
- Blood and circulatory problems: allergies, auto- immune disorders, cholesterol, diabetes, low and high blood pressure, toxemia, fibroids, endometriosis.

10.5   Ways to detox your body

No	Ways to detox	Solutions
1	Choose the right food	Opt for organic vegetables andfruits to decrease the toxins in your body. Fast and processed food which increase toxins should be avoided
2	Drink healthy clean water	Your body needs water to produce saliva, helps with perspiration and removes waste from the body.
3	Exercise regularly	Exercise helps you sweat, and sweating helps to release toxins through your skin
4	Purify the air you breathe	Keep your home air fresh and toxin-free, with a high-quality air purification device or house plants, like aloe -vera plants
5	Follow a diet pattern	There are many foods that aid detoxification- garlic, lemon, broccoli sprouts, mung beans, and raw vegetables.
6	Cleanse your body regularly	A complete body detox is a step-by- step that focuses on removing harmful organisms, chemicals, and toxic metals, while cleansing your colon, liver and kidneys.

Table 4

Sweating toxins out of the body is a great way to get rid of them either by exercise or with saunas. The lymph system drains toxins from the space between cells and is dependent on exercise to eliminate them.

Skin brushing is also considered beneficial to detoxification. Dead skin cells can block pores, preventing toxins elimination through the skin. Skin brushing should be done on dry skin and then followed by a bath to open the pores and allow toxins to come out.

"There is a long list of chronic diseases caused by toxin build up in our

bodies. The good news is that chronic diseases caused by lifestyle can be cured and respond positively to correct detoxification and nutrition".

Juicing-for-health.com   *Detoxification:*
An Introduction to Body Cleansing in Detoxification

Questions

1. Do you detox your body regularly and how often?

2. What do you use to detox?

3. Is food used or other means?

4. How do you feel when you detox?

5. Do you benefit from the detox process?

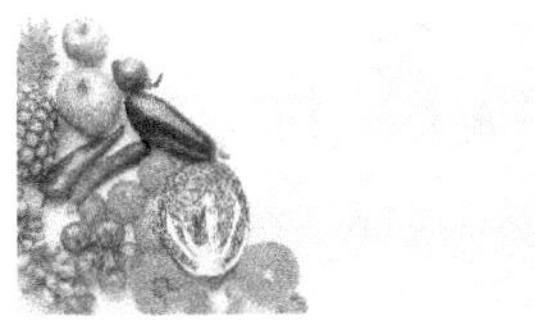

CHAPTER 11

Different Health Conditions

Nutrition has been around since the genesis of time. People had all they needed to eat healthily and to heal different types of diseases. Such common diseases are stated below:

11.1   Hay Fever:

What is hay fever?

It is an allergic inflammation of the nasal airways with symptoms mimicking a cold or flu but without the fever or high temperature. It is also the allergic reaction to pollen in the air. The number of people with this ailment has increased and more people suffer especially during spring and summer months.

Top tips:

To increase resistance and reduce symptoms, incorporate foods rich in antioxidants, such as vitamins A, B5, C and E, beta-carotene, selenium and zinc.

Take Amino acid l-methionine combined (500g) with calcium (400g), to increase its bioavailability and absorption, twice a day is an effective antihistamine. Amino acid is contained in high methionine foods like nuts, beef, lamb, cheese, turkey, pork, fish, shellfish, soy, eggs, dairy and beans. All these different types of food to be eaten which contain vitamins, minerals and other nutrients were discussed in chapter 2.

Other remedies include herbal tea, chamomile tea, ginger tea, peppermint tea and green tea.

Nutritional advice:

Eat a lot of antioxidant rich foods such as fruits and vegetables.

Eat seeds and nuts that are rich in selenium and zinc.

Limit or completely avoid gluten, dairy products and alcohol.

There are different types of hypertension but only one is discussed here. Others such as pulmonary hypertension is discussed in another series.

11.2   Hypertension (high blood pressure)

Hypertension or high blood pressure occurs when the pressure of blood being pumped through the arteries is higher than it should be.

Blood pressure is set by:

- Cardiac output: - the amount of blood pumped by each ventricle in one minute.

- Peripheral resistance: - the resistance that the heart must overcome to make the blood flow through the blood vessels of your circulatory system. The higher the blood pressure gets, the more difficult it takes the heart to pump the blood to the rest of the body.

- Stress: - the narrowing and thickening of arteries, arterial tension or thicker blood can produce high blood pressure.

- If left untreated, high blood pressure increases the risk of a heart attack or stroke

The only way of knowing there is a problem is to have your blood pressure checked.

Top Tips:

- Arterial tension is controlled by the balance of calcium, magnesium, and potassium in relation to sodium.

- Losing weight, avoiding alcohol, exercise and sleep can help reduce hypertension.

- Vitamin C and E and fish oils high in EPA and DHA (omega 3) helps to keep the blood thin.

Nutritional Advice:

- Follow a healthy nutritious diet, rich in potassium, calcium, magnesium, Vitamin C and E.

- Avoid excessive amounts of salt.

- Increase the intake of fruits - at least 5 a day.

- Increase the intake of vegetables that are rich in potassium, also aubergines are known to be beneficial for treating high blood pressure.

- Take a teaspoon of ground seeds a day as a source of extra calcium and magnesium and you may also try bitter melon.

- For Omega 3, eat fish about three times a week (not canned). Especially tuna, salmon not smoked, herring, or mackerel.

Remember everyone is different. As it's said, *"one man's meat is another man's poison."* I may eat a fruit or vegetable and feel in optimal health, whilst another person may react. Therefore, it is important to listen to your own body.

11.3   The Heart

The heart is responsible for the function of the blood flow in the body, the arteries and veins. The blood vessels are part of the system and these are the means through which the blood is carried around the body. Every organ in the body needs blood, it is the lifeline of the whole body and human beings.

If the heart malfunctions, then the whole body would suffer from **High Blood Pressure** because the heart is not working properly. Our Creator created a solution for every organ and part of the body, we need to go back to Genesis in the Bible and find out what they are. I have put together some information about the certain diseases that are common with people living with sickle cell anaemia. Many solutions can be traced back to eating good nutrition.

Diet may impact the way blood flows through the body. An acidic diet while overworking the body's buffer system, is also likely to be high in cholesterol, saturated fat and trans-fat. This would impair blood circulation in the long-term. It is noted that the daily ***Dietary Approaches to Stop Hypertension (DASH)*** diet shares many similarities to an alkaline diet. One of the main functions of blood is to transport oxygen and nutrition to the cells and one of the principal benefits of correct body pH balance is the body's ability to transfer oxygen efficiently through the body. This is vital for immunity and high-energy living.

DASH Diet Foods for High Blood Pressure (Hypertension) (webmd.com)

THE HEART

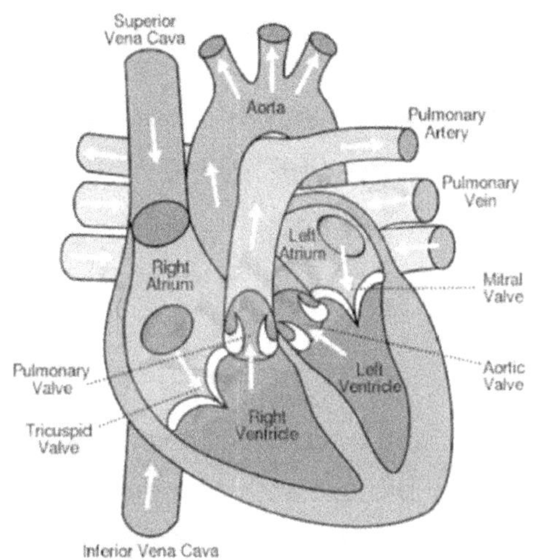

www.sciencekids.co.nz/pictures/humanbody/heartdiagram.html

11.4   Blood Disorders and Anaemia

• Blood

"Our blood is miraculous in all that it accomplishes for our body, it is the river of life. Blood has three main functions to provide:

- o   Life
- o   Health
- o   Protection

The red blood cells transport oxygen from the lungs to every area of the body. They also disperse nutrients and vitamins to the exact parts of the body where they are needed; our body's very own 'Amazon Prime.'

The white blood cells, along with lymphocytes, help to build the body's entire immune system. Each cell in the blood has particular tasks they perform, helping the body strengthen itself and fight off foreign invaders that could make us ill. Some cells build up the immune system while others help the immune system to know exactly what invaders to target. There are certain cells that recognise an invasive organism so that the immune system can respond quicker the next time it encounters that same organism. There are other cells that keep the immune system under control so that it doesn't start attacking the good cells within our bodies. What a glorious army the Lord created within us, sustaining and protecting our bodies with this complex combination of blood cells.

Furthermore, the immune system is like an engine in our body, it fixes or gets rid of infections and diseases, if you do not take care of it, the body will begin to attract different diseases, infections and the body becomes run down.

When we get a chance to study the intricate ways our bodies were created, it gives insight into our walk with the Lord. He is so intentional. So it is no accident that blood plays such an integral role in the Bible. *"There is life in the blood. It's not just a catchphrase."*

(i)   *Johnson, Beni. The Power of Communion (p. 30-31)*
(ii)   *Destiny Image, Inc. Kindle Edition.*

• **Anaemia**

"Anaemia is a condition where the body has insufficient healthy red blood cells to carry enough oxygen to the organs and the body tissues." There are different types of anaemia, each has its own cause.

Iron is needed to make haemoglobin which is a key part of blood formation responsible for the delivery of oxygen and other nutrients to our tissues, brain, muscles and organs. When there is insufficient blood these organs suffer damage which is dangerous to the body as a whole. If a person is lacking in iron, it means they are not producing sufficient red blood cells. Therefore, the person becomes pale in appearance.

Most blood cells including red blood cells are produced regularly in the bone marrow - a spongy material found within the cavities of large bones; to produce haemoglobin and red blood cells, the body needs iron, vitamin B-12, folate and other nutrients from the foods you eat.

The body makes three types of blood cells - white blood cells to fight infection, platelets to help blood clot and red blood cells to carry oxygen throughout your body. Red blood cells contain haemoglobin - an iron-rich protein that gives blood its red colour. Haemoglobin enables red blood cells to carry oxygen from the lungs to all parts of the body and to carry carbon dioxide from other parts of the body to the lungs to be exhaled.

Most blood cells, including red blood cells, are produced regularly in the bone marrow — a spongy material found within the cavities of large bones. To produce haemoglobin and red blood cells, the body needs iron, vitamin B-12, folate and other nutrients from foods consumed."

Types of Anaemia and Their Causes Include:

- **Iron deficiency anaemia:** - This is the most common type of anaemia worldwide. Iron deficiency anaemia is caused by a shortage of iron in the body. Bone marrow needs iron to make haemoglobin. Without adequate iron, the body would not produce enough haemoglobin for red blood cell formation.

  This type of anaemia occurs in many   pregnant women, it is also caused by blood loss such as from heavy menstrual bleeding, an ulcer, cancer and regular use of some over-the-counter pain relievers especially aspirin. With the right type of nutrition and supplements would provide the basic solution.

- **Vitamin deficiency anaemia:** - In addition to iron, the body needs folate and vitamin B-12 to produce enough healthy red blood cells. A diet lacking in these and other key nutrients can cause decreased red blood cell production. Additionally, some people may consume enough B-12 but their bodies aren't able to process the vitamin. This can lead to vitamin deficiency anaemia also known as *pernicious anaemia*.

- **Anaemia of chronic disease:** - Certain diseases - such as cancer, HIV/AIDS, rheumatoid arthritis, kidney disease, Crohn's disease and other chronic inflammatory diseases can interfere with the production of red blood cells.

- **Aplastic anaemia: -** This rare, life-threatening anaemia occurs when the body doesn't produce sufficient red blood cells. Causes of aplastic anaemia include infections, certain medicines, autoimmune diseases and exposure to toxic chemicals.

- **Anaemias associated with bone marrow disease: -** A variety of diseases such as leukaemia and myelofibrosis, can cause anaemia by affecting blood production in the bone marrow. The effects of these types of cancer and cancer-like disorders vary from mild to life-threatening.

- **Haemolytic anaemias: -** This group of anaemia develops when red blood cells are destroyed faster than bone marrow replaces them. Certain blood diseases increase red blood cell destruction. Haemolytic anaemia can be inherited or can be developed later in life.

- **Sickle cell anaemia: -** This serious condition is an inherited hemolytic anaemia. It is caused by a defective form of haemoglobin that forces red blood cells to assume an abnormal crescent (sickle) shape. These irregular blood cells die prematurely, resulting in a chronic shortage of red blood cells.

- **Other anaemias: -** There are several other forms of anaemia, such as thalassemia and malarial anaemia.

Mayo Clinic

https://www.mayoclinic.org/diseases-conditions/anemia/symptoms-_causes/syc-20351360

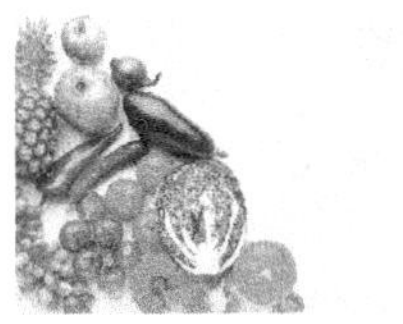

CHAPTER 12

Sickle Cell Anaemia (part 1)

"Sickle cell disease results from a single genetic mutation that causes a person's red blood cells to form an abnormal, sickle shape. These sickled cells can clog the blood vessels and deprive cells of oxygen. In turn, this lack of oxygen wreaks havoc on the body, damaging organs, causing severe pain and potentially leading to premature death."

NIH launches initiative to accelerate genetic therapies to cure sickle cell disease on the September 13, 2018, 8:00 AM EDT

Emphasis has been laid on nutrition and its importance to sickle cell disease but would continue in the next series. Below is an extract from a journal, which may be referred to as it is a research in nutrition on sickle cell. I believe that nutrition plays an important part in lesser crisis and the maintenance of the cells of the body with sickle cell anaemia.

1. Nutrient insufficiencies/deficiencies

According to the journal below, nutritional intake in Sickle cell patients has been found to be quite poor and this situation needs to be corrected.

Many of the complications associated with Sickle cell disease such as growth retardation, delayed sexual maturity and a weak immune system could be considered partly due to nutritional deficiencies.

2. Role of macronutrient deficiencies

It was reported that supplementation of a high protein diet, resulted in decreased infection in children with Sickle Cell Anaemia.

Arginine supplementation through exogenous sources can restore low global arginine bioavailability (GAB). Arginine supplementation is quite successful in treating patients with leg ulcer, pulmonary hypertension and pain.

3.   Role of micronutrients

"Zinc supplementation to pre pubertal aged sickle cell anaemia patients were found to be beneficial on their linear growth and weight. Zinc sulphate has been found quite effective in reducing RBC's dehydration. It was also found to reduce sickle cell crises, pain and other life-threatening complications. Zinc supplementation not only improved growth and weight of SCD children but also gave a boost to their immune system by offering antibacterial protection thereby making it's supplementation essential".

4.   Role of vitamins

As compared to their peers, SCD children are known to show decreased height and weight resulting in poor growth. Blood deficiency of several vitamins such as A, B6, B12, C, D, E and minerals like Zinc, Magnesium is observed in patients with SCD by many researchers which are the most contributing factors towards their poor growth and weight.

All these vitamins and minerals contribute to the good health of those with sickle cell disease. For more information, please read the health journal below:

Precipitating factors and targeted therapies in combating the perils of sickle cell disease--- A special nutritional consideration Nutrition & Metabolism201613:50 *https://doi.org/10.1186/s12986-016-0109-7 Published: 8 August 2*

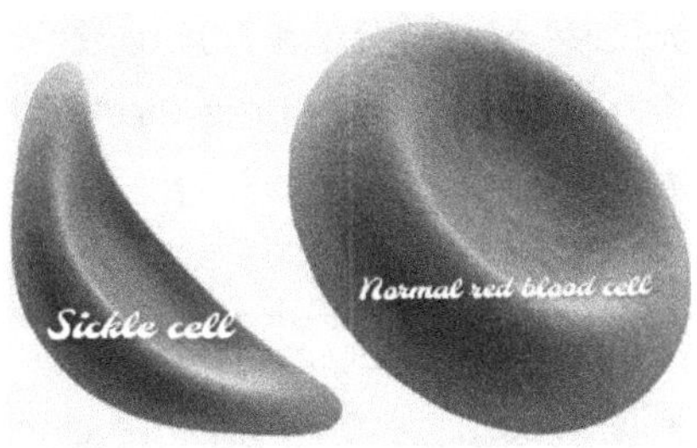

This picture shows the difference between the sickle cell disease blood shape and that of a normal cell blood shape.

Nutritional Advice:

- Red meat is one of the good sources of iron but it is rich in saturated fat.

- Other sources that do not have high fat as meat are eggs, spinach, kale, beans, lentils, prunes, dried apricot, molasses, pumpkin seeds, pumpkin leaves and bitter leaf.

- Most of these are rich in Folic acid which is needed for the body.

- Vitamin B12 is naturally found in animal products like fish, meat, chicken, eggs and milk products.

- All these are foods that would help to build the immune system and improve the hemoglobin in blood making it rich again.

https://www.mayoclinic.org/diseases-conditions/anemia/symptoms.../syc-20351360

General Advice:

Important things to note for those with sickle cell are: -

- Always listen to your body, it will tell you what is going on and how it feels, whether tired, hot or cold.

- Stay hydrated by drinking alkaline water, this is very important if your body is too acidic, it lowers your immune system and you start picking up infections.

- Make sure you are not stressed but relax most of the time, too much stress brings on a crisis. As I mentioned in the beginning God is the author and finisher of our faith. He is always ready to listen to us.

As a young child, my mother made sure she cooked a lot of vegetables like bitter leaves, pumpkin leaves and other types of rich vegetables. This was due to the fact that I was anaemic most of the time because I had sickle cell disease. But all these vegetables were made fresh most of the time, I had to drink the juice from the bitter leaf plant *(very bitter)*. However, it was extremely beneficial for my body. I noticed that with all these nutrients; I was becoming healthier each day.

CONCLUSION

On my journey to good health, I realized that proper nutrition, hydration, sleep and exercise are essential. Sleep plays an important role because when we sleep properly our body tends to repair and heal itself. Most diseases are healed and the body becomes whole again.

In my experience, nutrition was the path I had to walk and by the grace of God I am alive, thriving and prosperous to fulfil God's divine purpose in my life. Good nutrition has been of immense importance to me and many others who were battling with various illnesses. It is not advisable to ignore the doctor's advice or refuse professionally prescribed medication or help; there is a place for each.

It is advisable to incorporate responsible practices into maintaining a healthy active lifestyle for wholesomeness and longevity. And more importantly, listen to the commands of God our Creator, who created every part of our body and how it works. Every plant and animal on this planet has a purpose; each organ and other parts of our body have a part to play.

It is highly advisable to adopt a practice of eating a healthy diet and praying to God for complete healing; for He knows all. If He created every plant and every other element for our survival, it can only follow that He can and indeed do the impossible.

Nourishing nutrition is a lifestyle which is greatly beneficial to adopt. By doing so, our immune system becomes strengthened, remains healthy and is well able to fight off any disease. We flourish when we enjoy optimum health. Our body being the temple of God; He has given us all we need to take care of it. However, the responsibility remains ours to do so. He knows our beginning, our end and everything in between. The same God who created life in us can be trusted with the details of our life.

In the series 2, I would continue with different health topics, watch out for this.

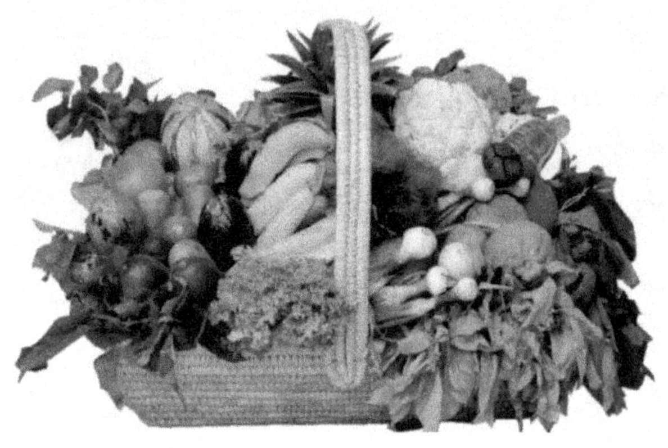

Nutritious Basket

REFERENCES

1. 23rd October 2019 by the NHLBI (National   Heart, Lung and Blood Institute)   www.nhlbi.nih.gov/health-topics/sickle-cell-disease

2. Sharecare – www.sharecare.com/health/nutrition- diet/articles

3. Neal yard How Food works DK pg 12, 13

4. A learning program devised by Byjus.   www.byjus.com

5. MedlinePlus- www.medlineplus.gov/ency/article/002458.htm

6. 15 Health Benefits of Avocado (ehealthzine.com) by Hezy Evans | April 20,

7. Finelib.com

8. www.sciencedirect.com

9. www.verywellhealth.com written 16/10/2020

10. www.medlineplus.gov -Medline plus - study of 19th Oct 2020 giving concerns of Covid 19

11. Neal's Yard- How food works from DK

12. Global healing centre: https://www.globalhealingcenter.com

13. www.medlineplus.gov

14. Dr. Christopher Vasey, Naturopathic Doctor in his book - The Water Prescription

15. By Roddy Macdonald Founder & Managing Director Of Water For Health

16. Smith, Laura Harris. The 30-Day Faith Detox (p. 21), Baker Publishing Group. Kindle Edition.

17. www.juicing-for-health.com

18. https://r.search.yahoo.com/_ylt=AwrlS.YhUAxhko0AUgl3Bwx.;_ylu=Y29s bwMEcG9zAzEEdnRpZANDMjAxN18xBHNlYwNzcg-- /RV=2/RE=1628225697/RO=10/RU=https%3a%2f%2fjuicing-for- health.com%2fdetoxification/RK=2/RS=Kgoz9ZYw4WPckdcekToae_Oc KmA-

19. Dietary Approaches to Stop Hypertension (DASH) DASH Diet Foods for High Blood Pressure (Hypertension) (webmd.com)

20. www.sciencekids.co.nz/pictures/humanbody/heartdiagram.html

21. Johnson, Beni. The Power of Communion (p. 30-31).

22. Destiny Image, Inc. Kindle Edition.

23. Mayo Clinic : https://www.mayoclinic.org/diseases-conditions/anemia/symptoms- causes/syc-20351360

24. NIH initiative - September 13, 2018, 8:00 AM EDT: Precipitating factors and targeted therapies in combating the perils of sickle cell disease--- A special nutritional consideration Nutrition & Metabolism201613:50 https://doi.org/10.1186/s12986-016-0109-7 Published: 8 August 2

25. https://www.mayoclinic.org/diseases-conditions/anemia/symptoms.../syc-20351360 Author: Shahida A . Khan, Ghazi Damanhouri. Published year 2016

26. https://www.tyndale.com

27. Scripture quotations marked (NLT) are taken from the Holy Bible, New Living Translation, copyright ©1996, 2004, 2015 by Tyndale House Foundation. Used by permission of Tyndale House Publishers, Carol Stream, Illinois 60188. All rights reserved.

28. https://www.thomasnelson.com

29. Scripture taken from the New King James Version®. Copyright © 1982 by Thomas Nelson. Used by permission. All rights reserved.

30. https://www.thepassiontranslation.com

31. Scripture quotations marked TPT are from The Passion Translation®. Copyright © 2017, 2018, 2020 by Passion & Fire Ministries, Inc. Used by permission. All rights reserved. ThePassionTranslation.com.